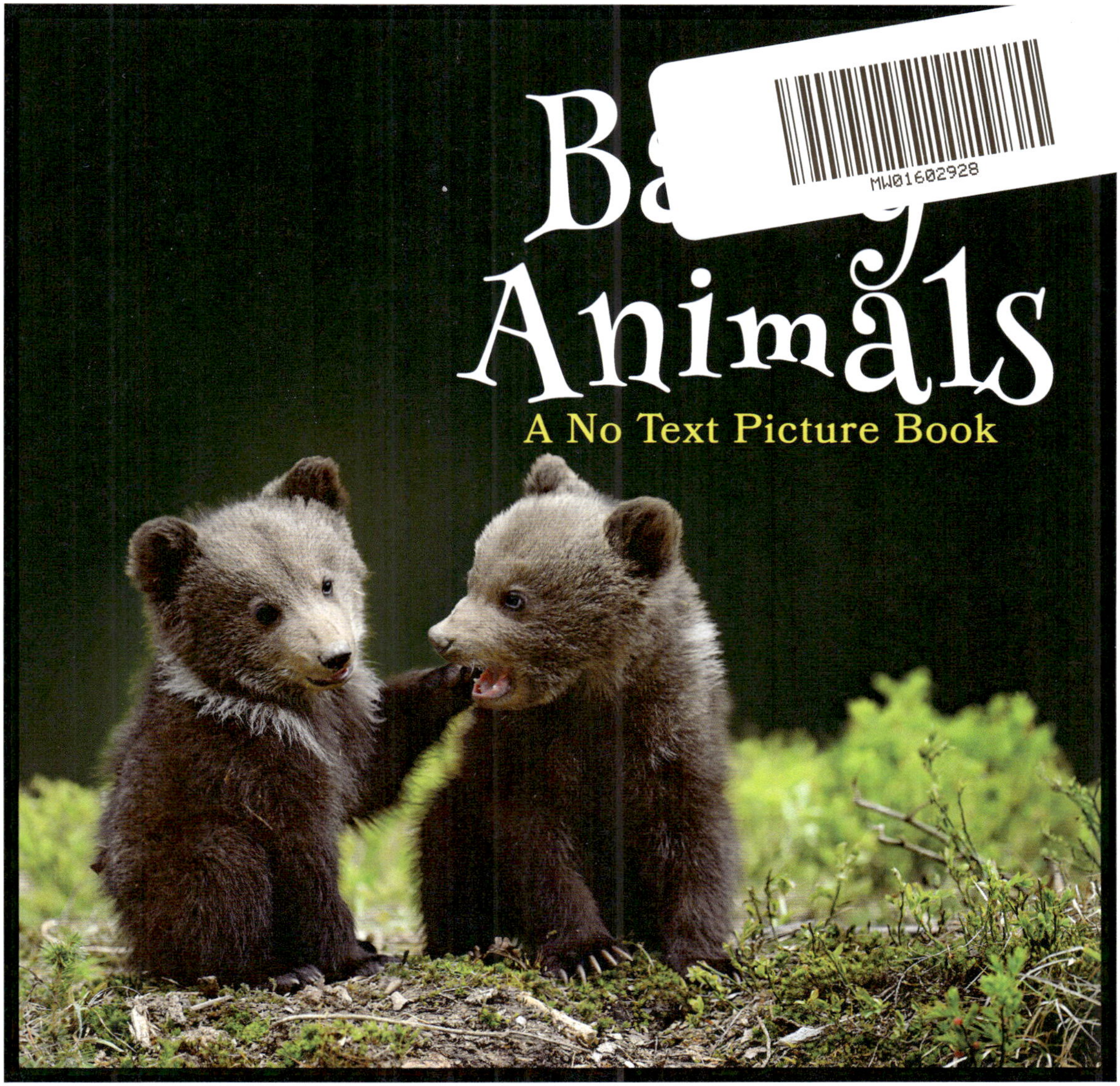

Baby Animals

A No Text Picture Book

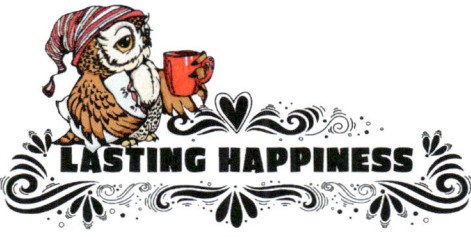

© 2021 Lasting Happiness | All rights reserved.
No part of this book may be reproduced or copied in any manner without prior written permission from the publisher.

ISBN: 9798708130129

To:

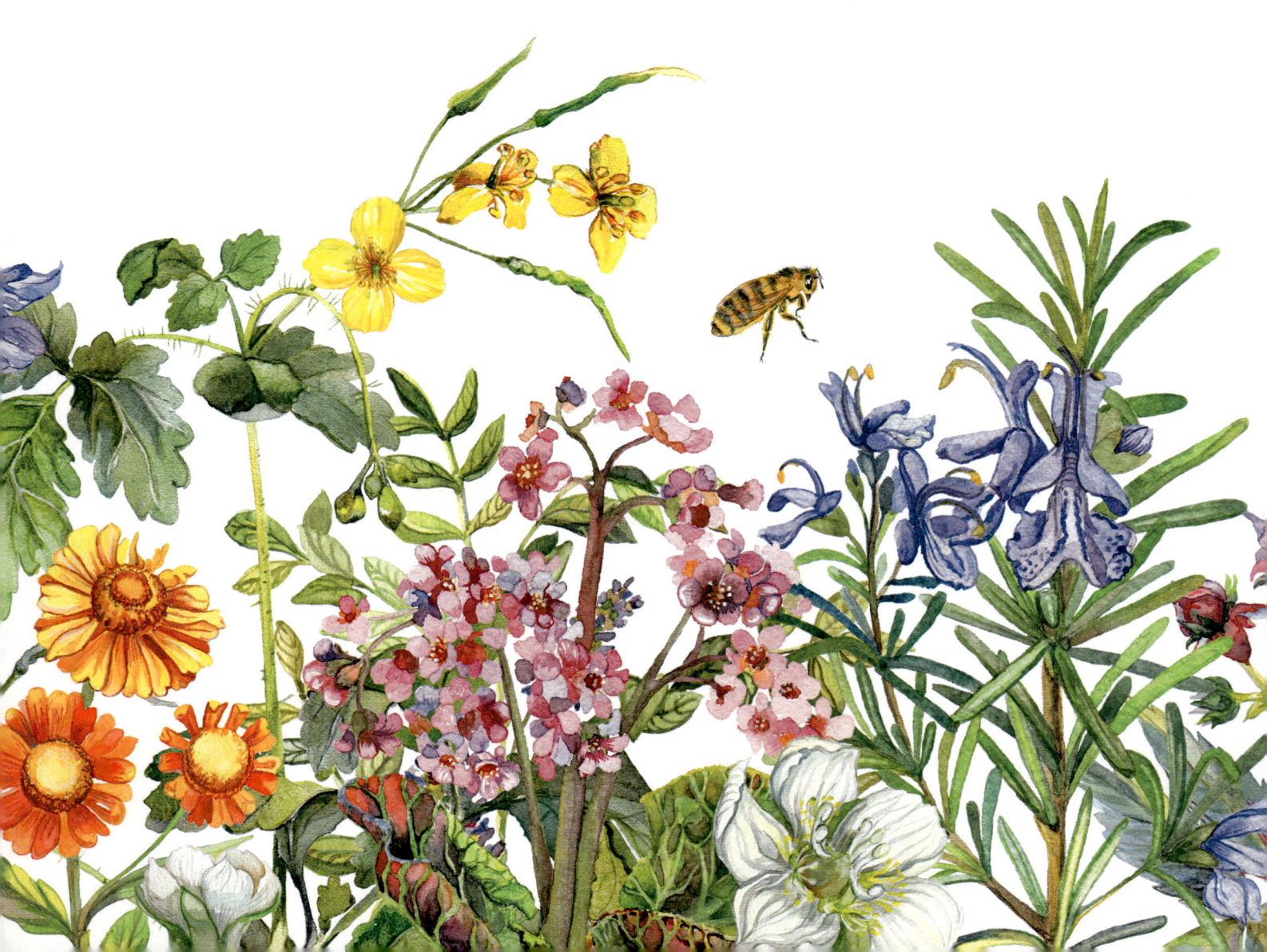

FROM:

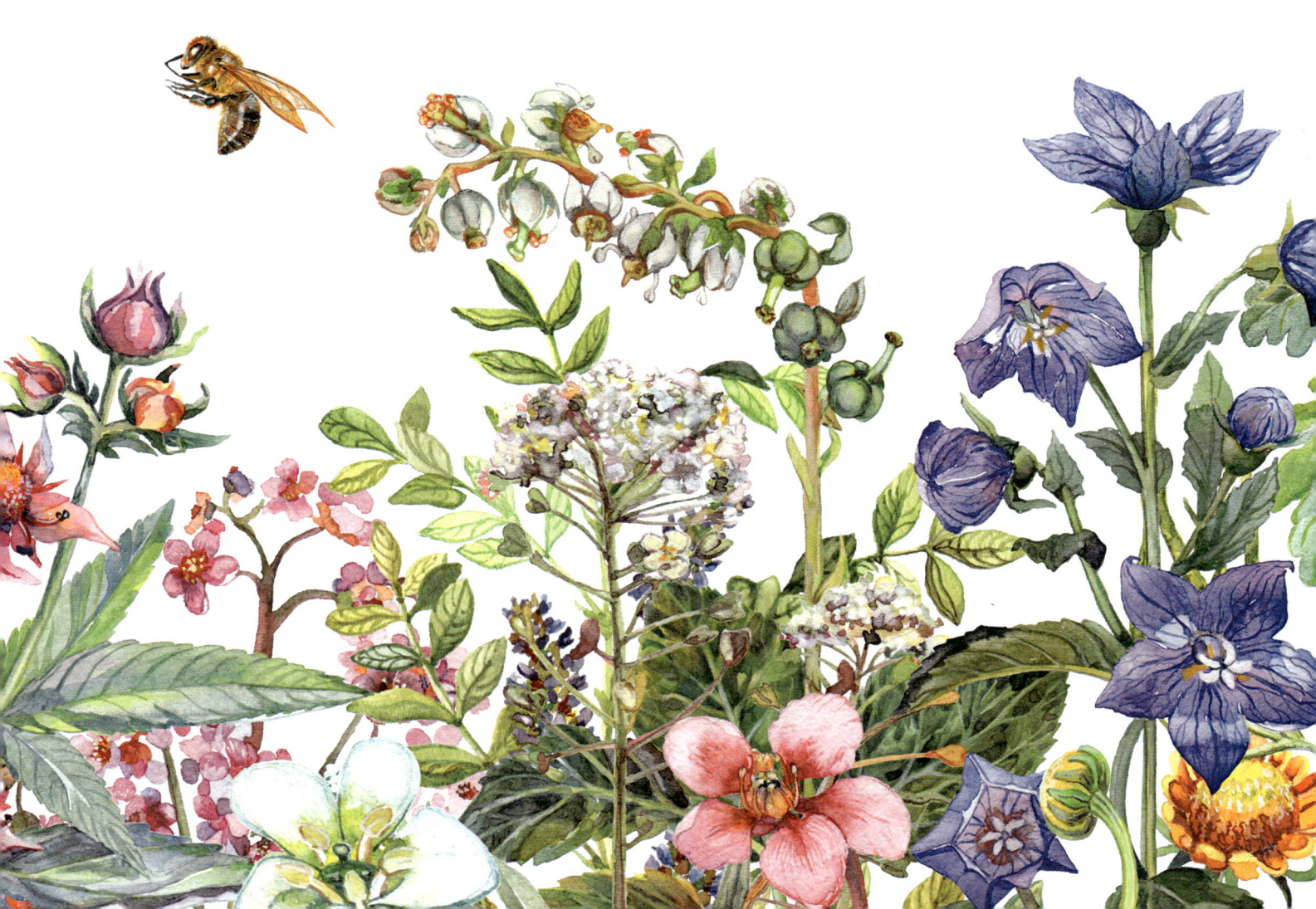

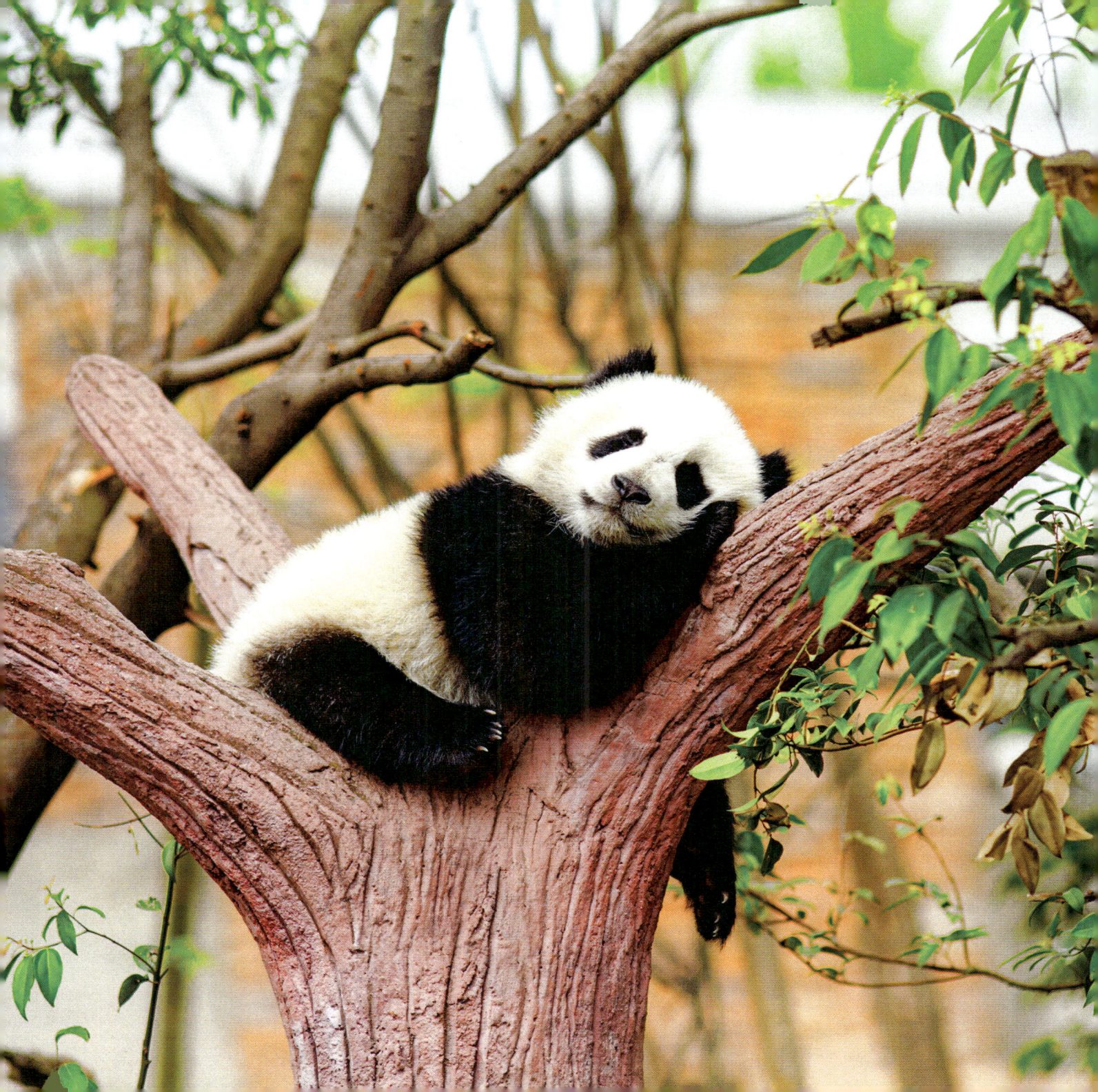

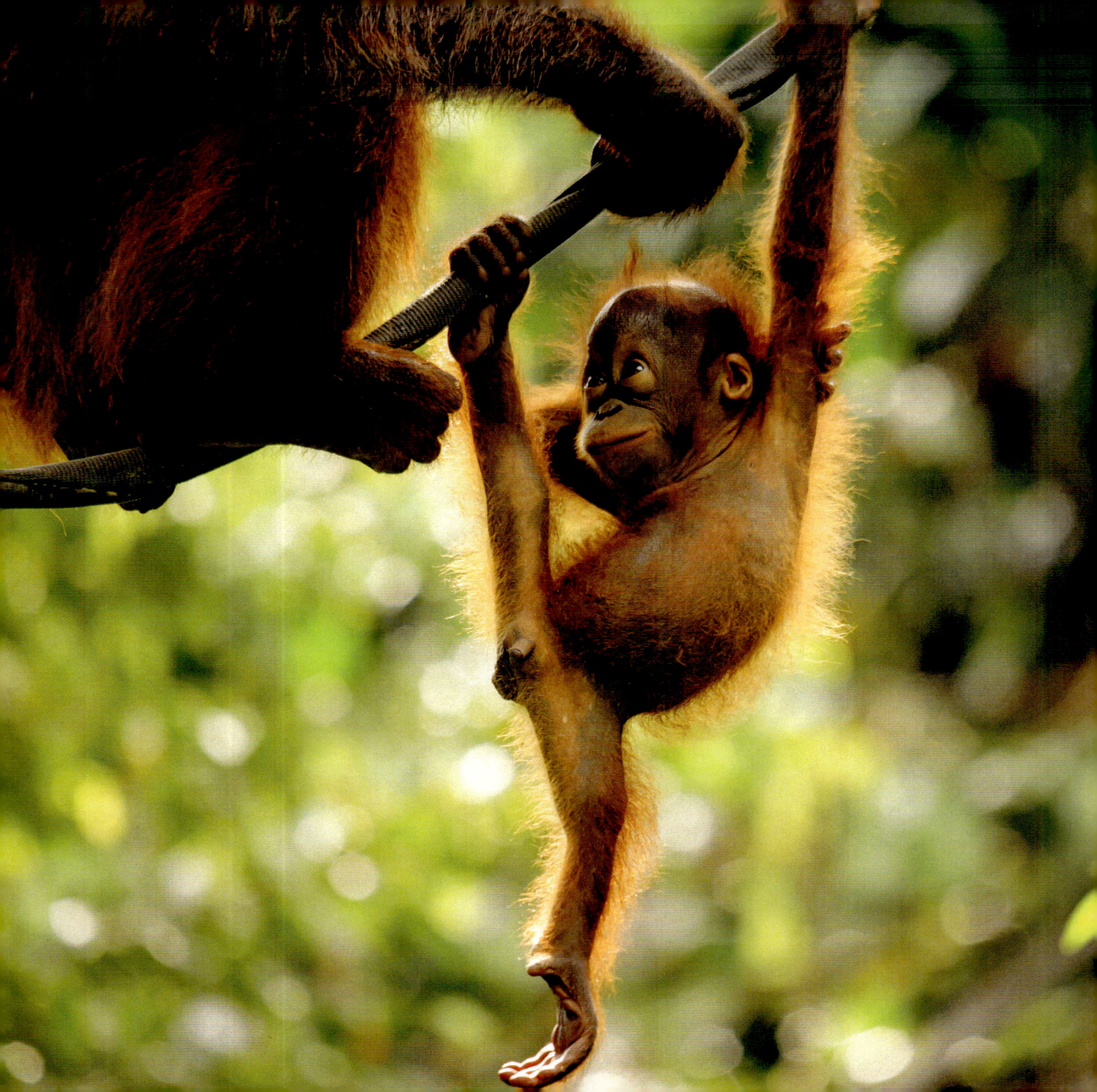

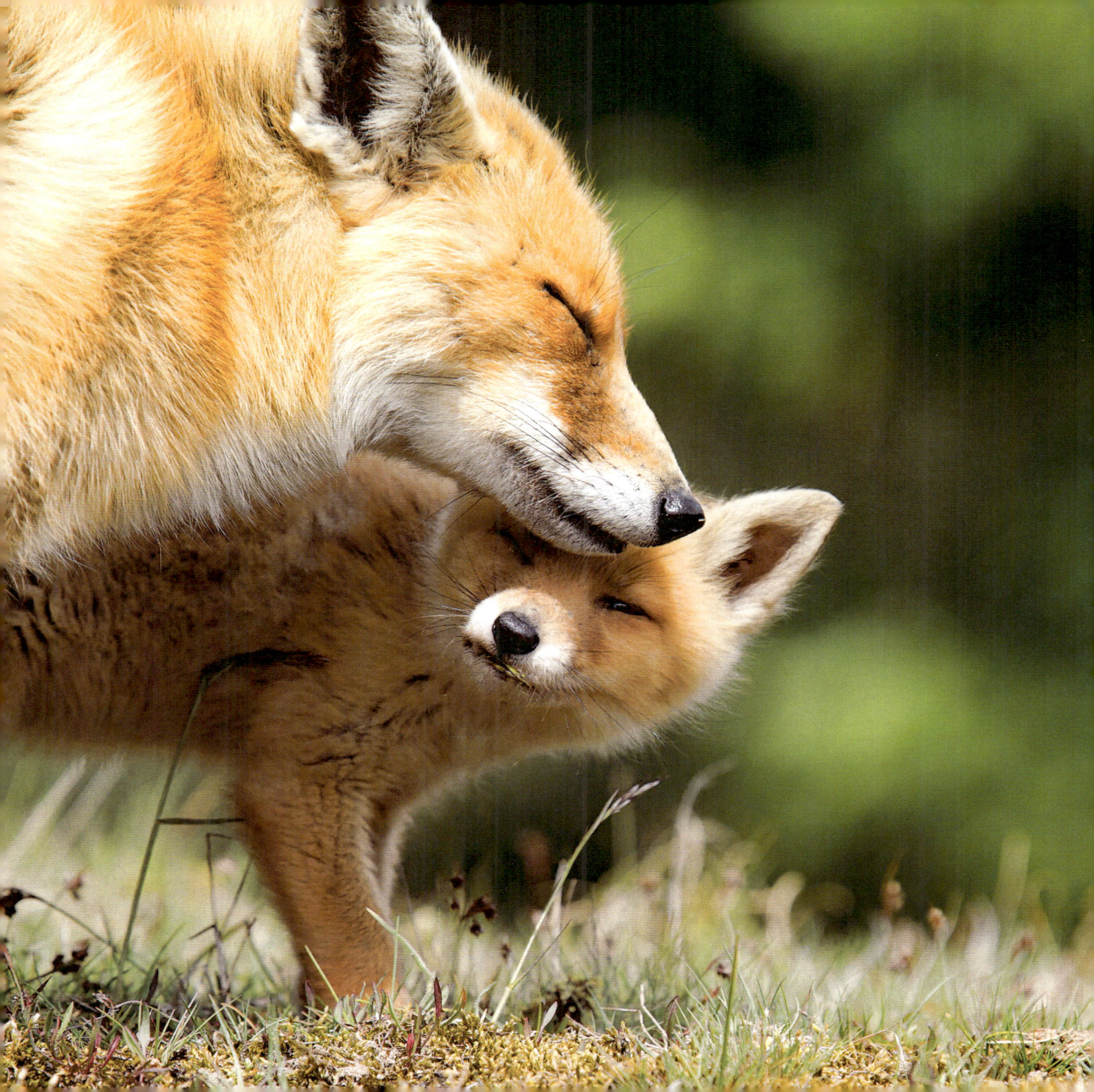

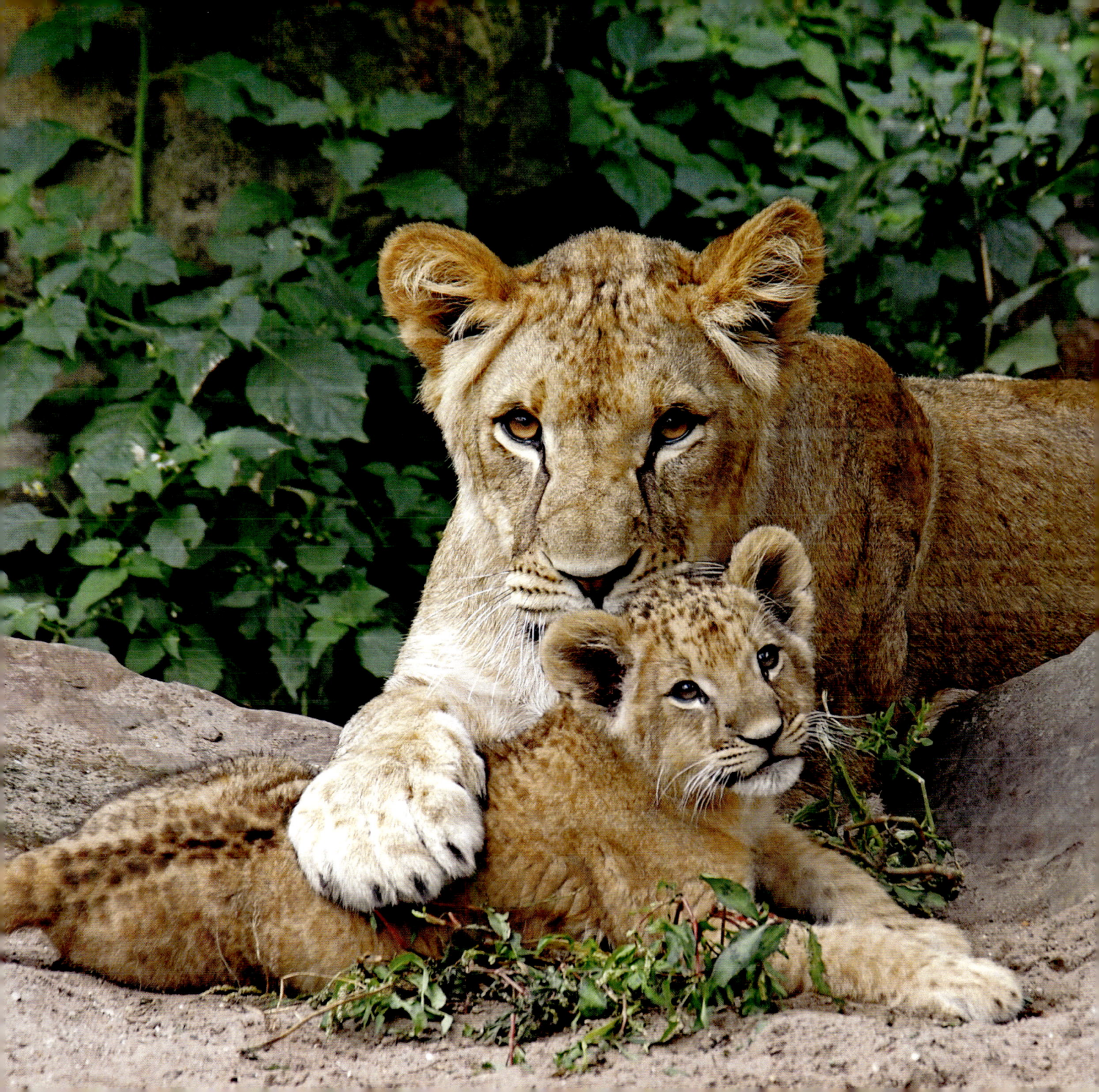

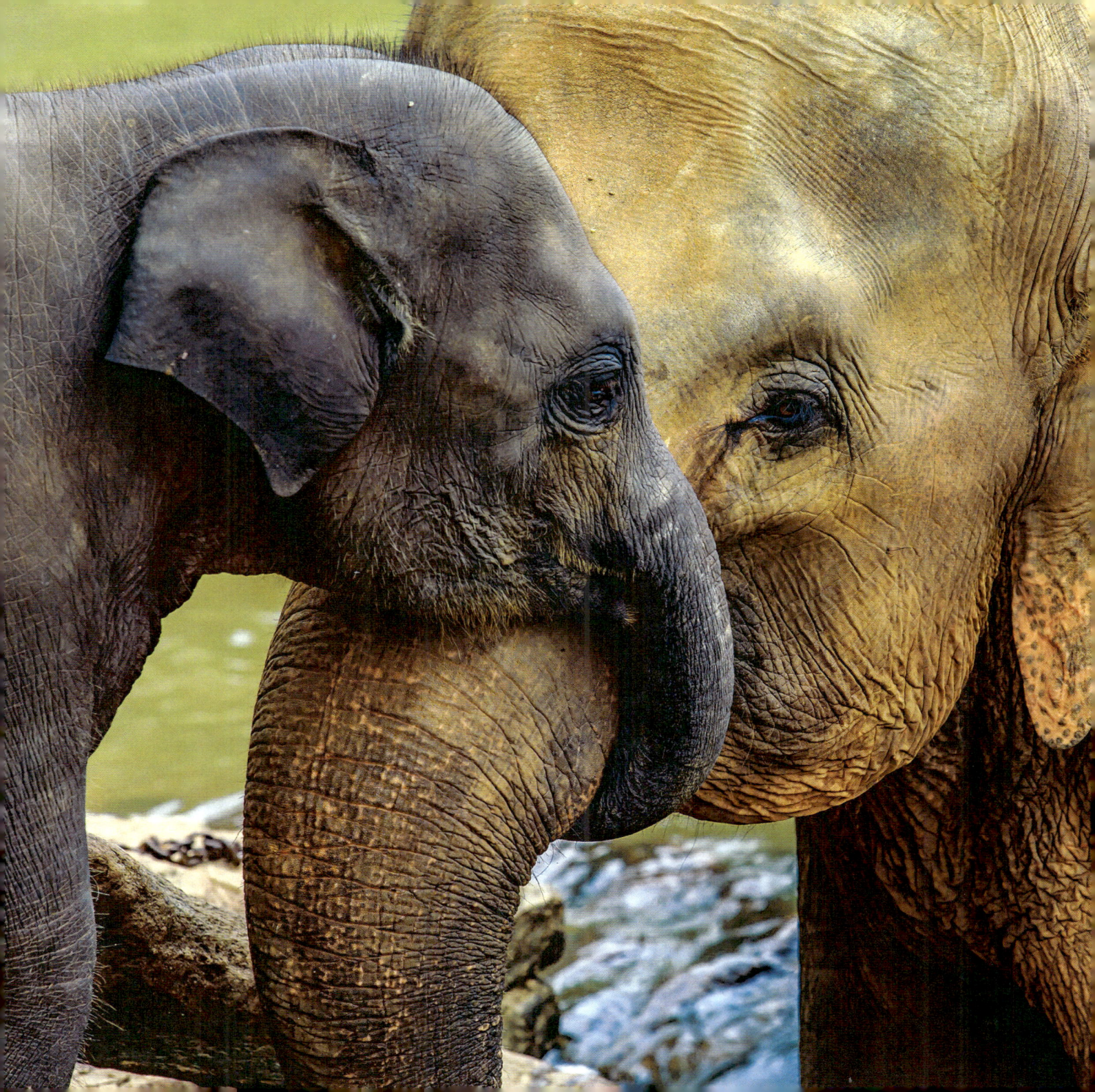

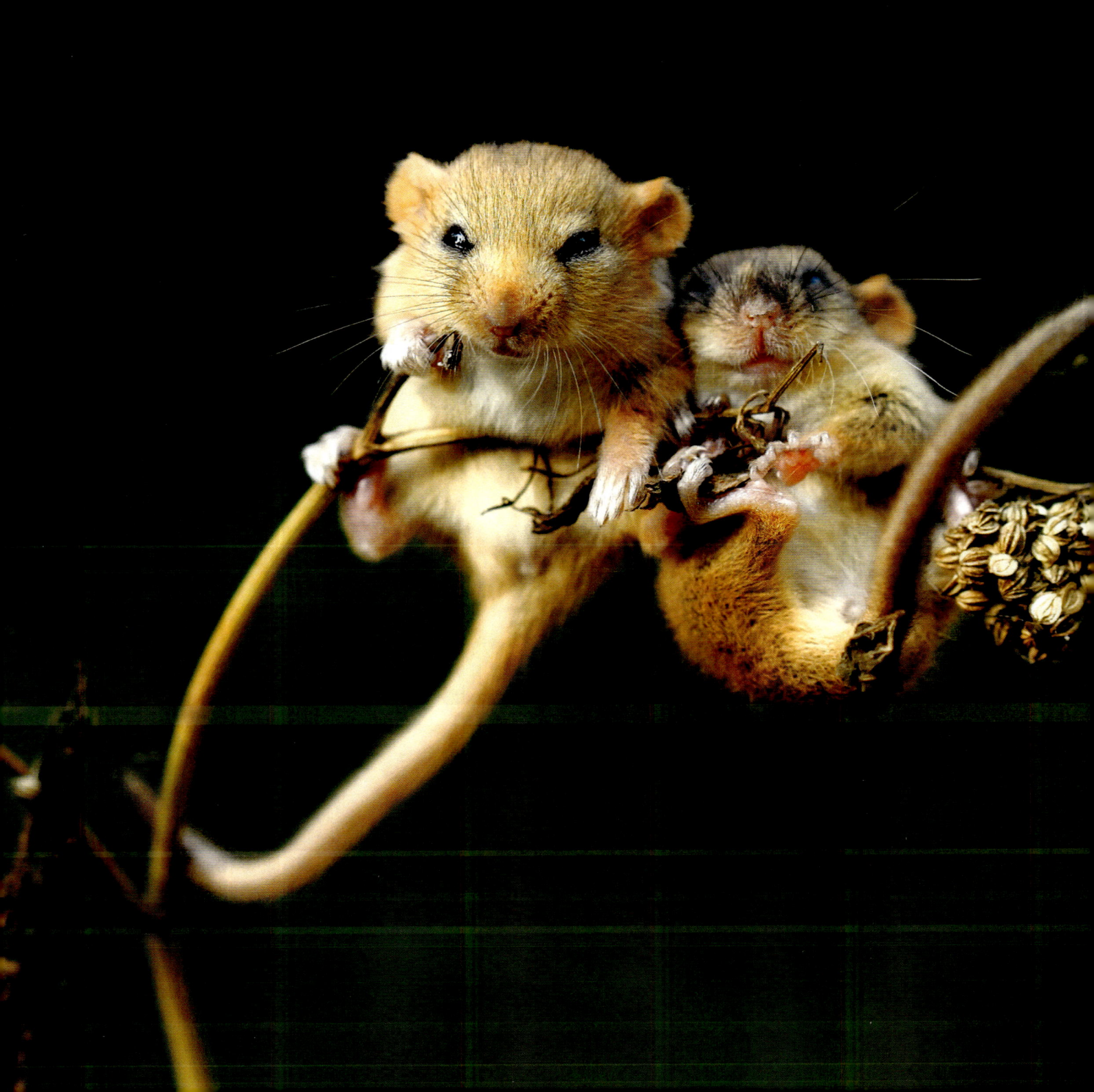

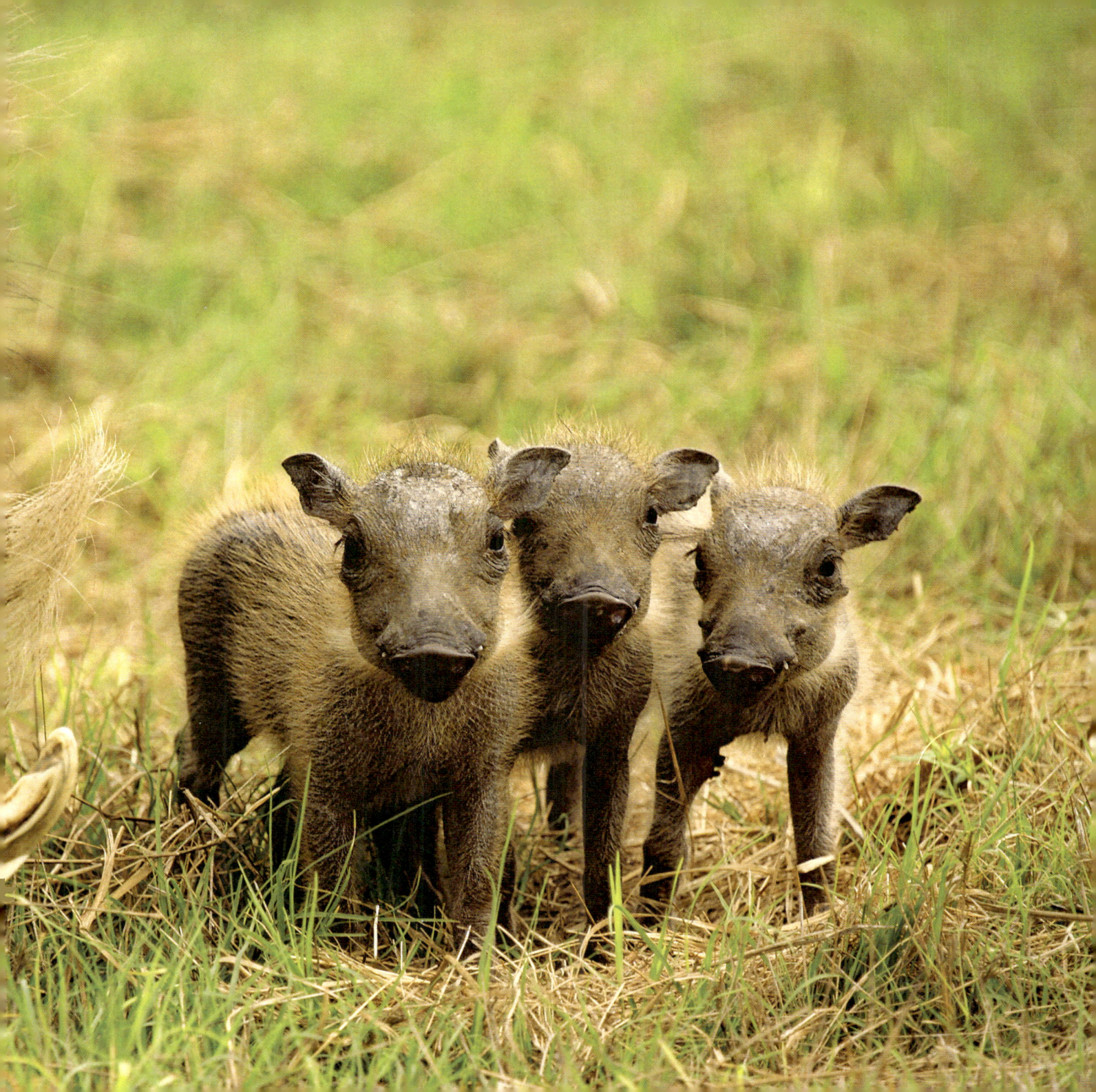

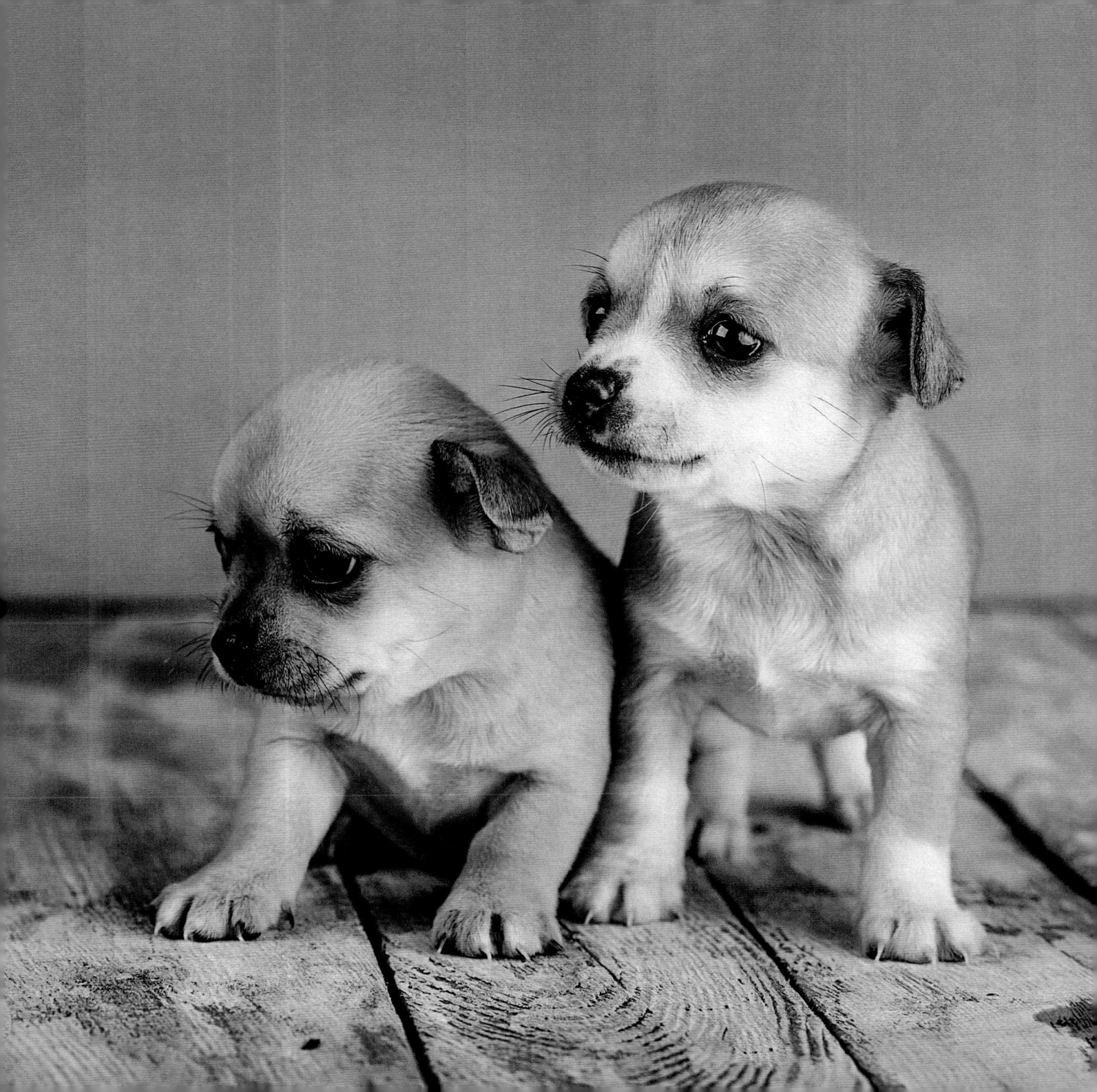

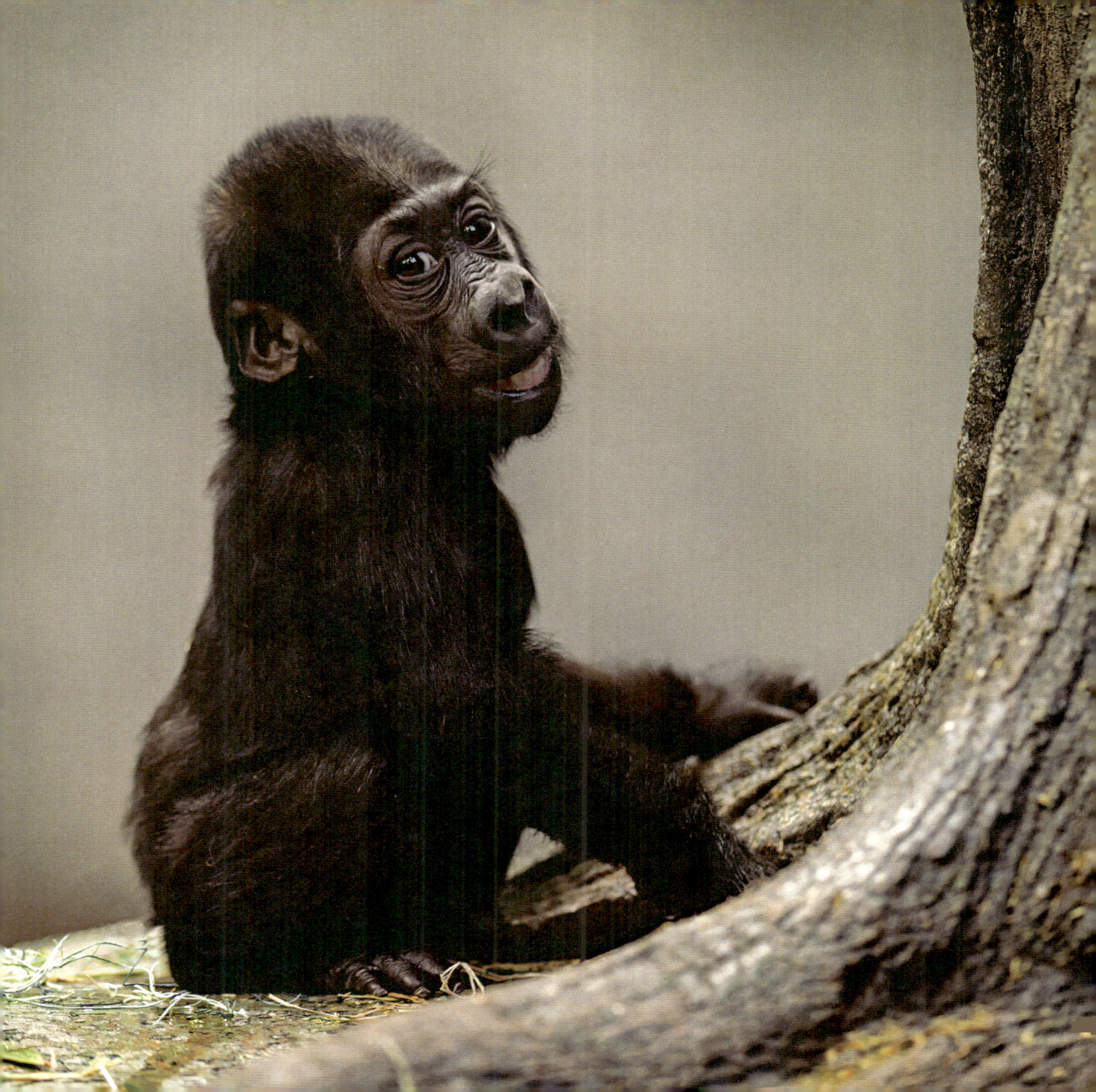

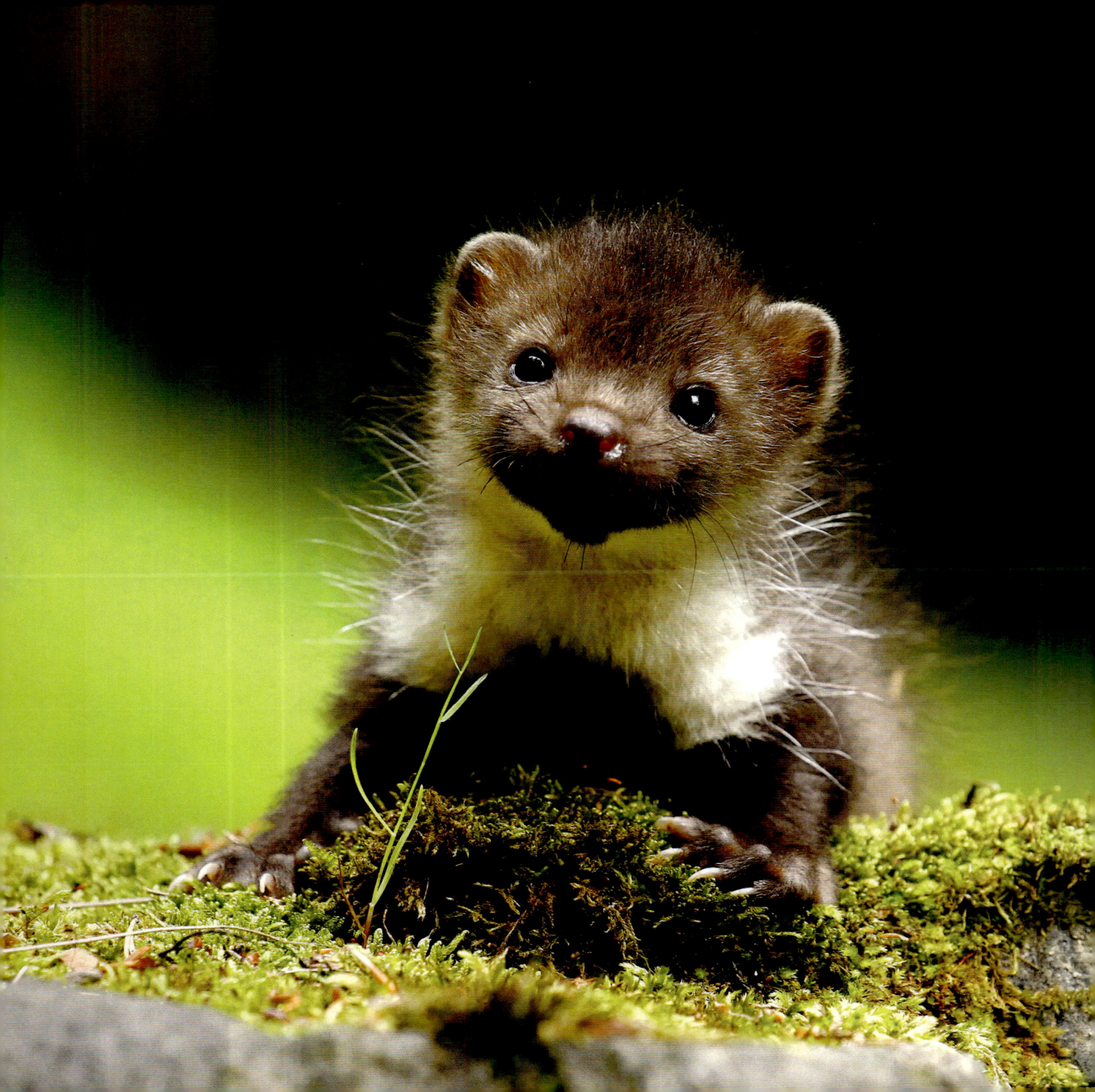

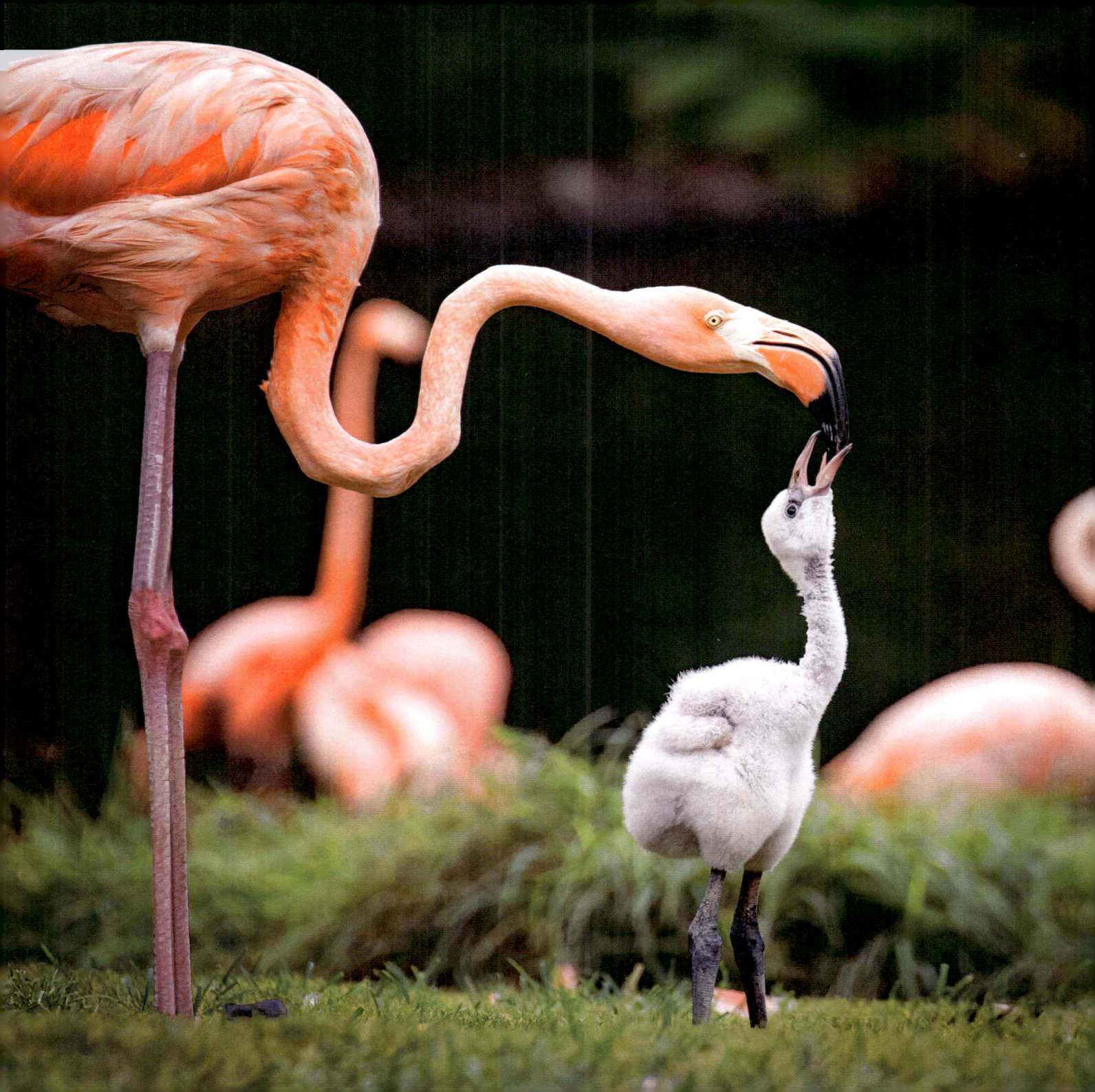

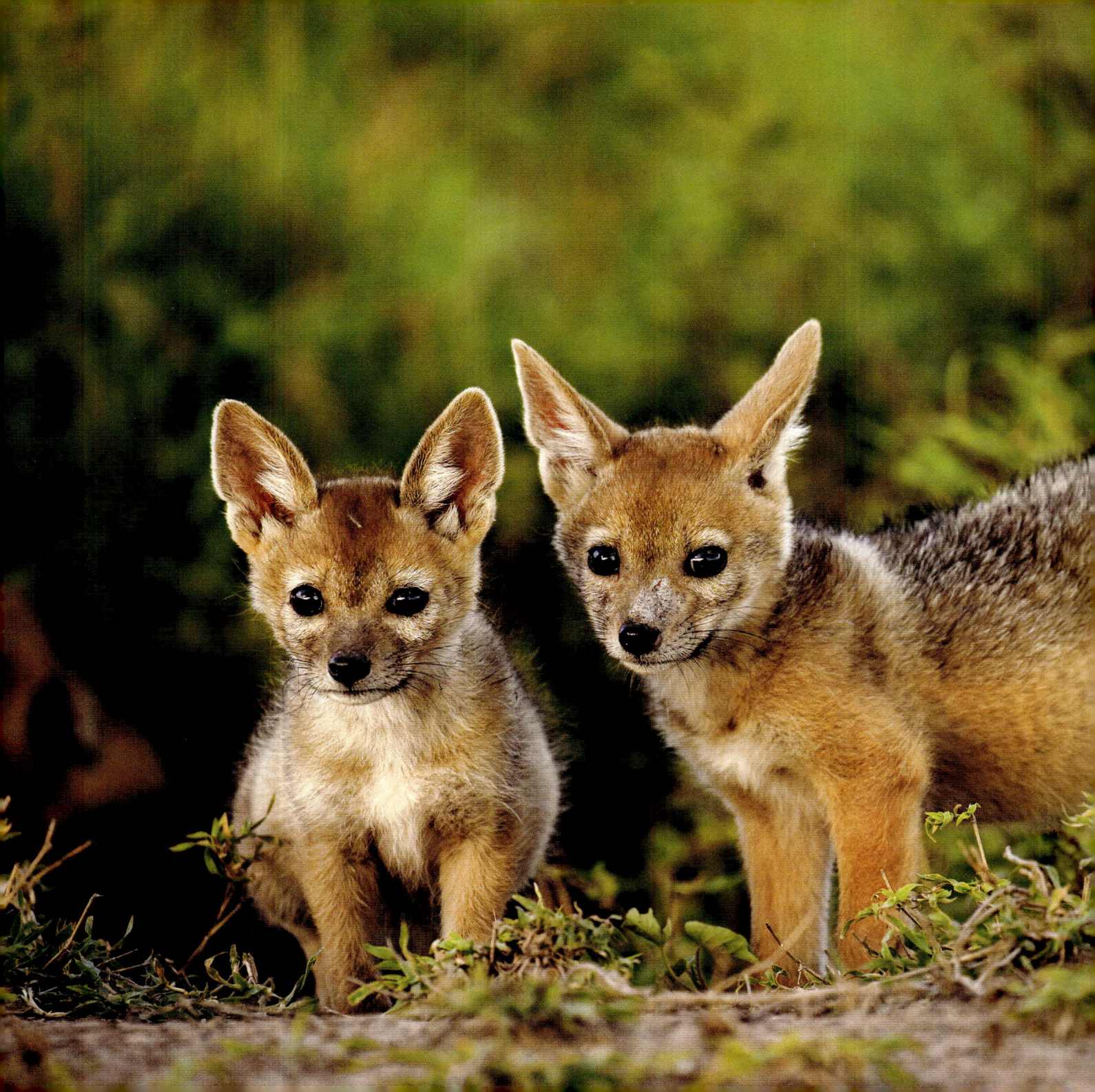

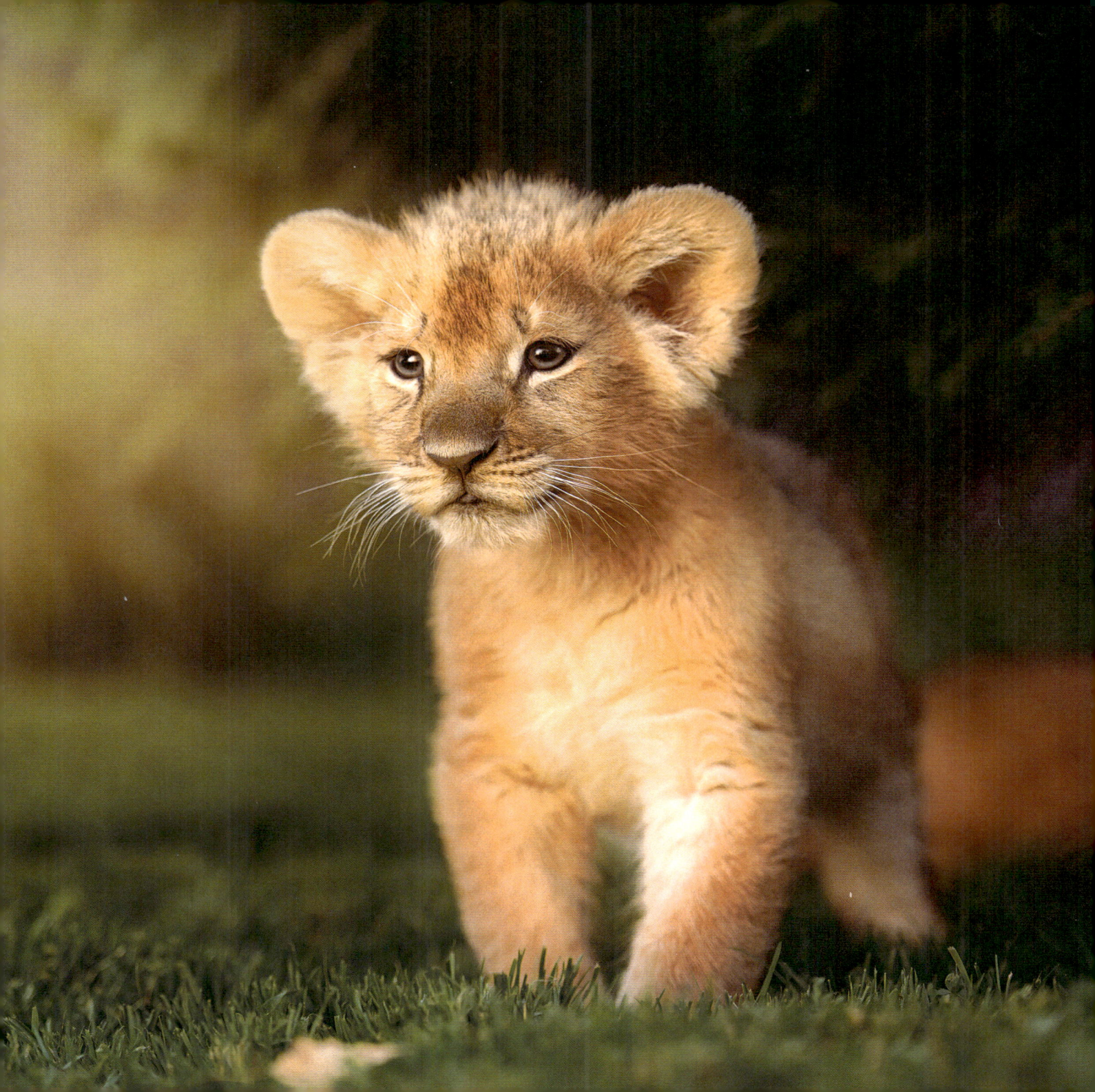

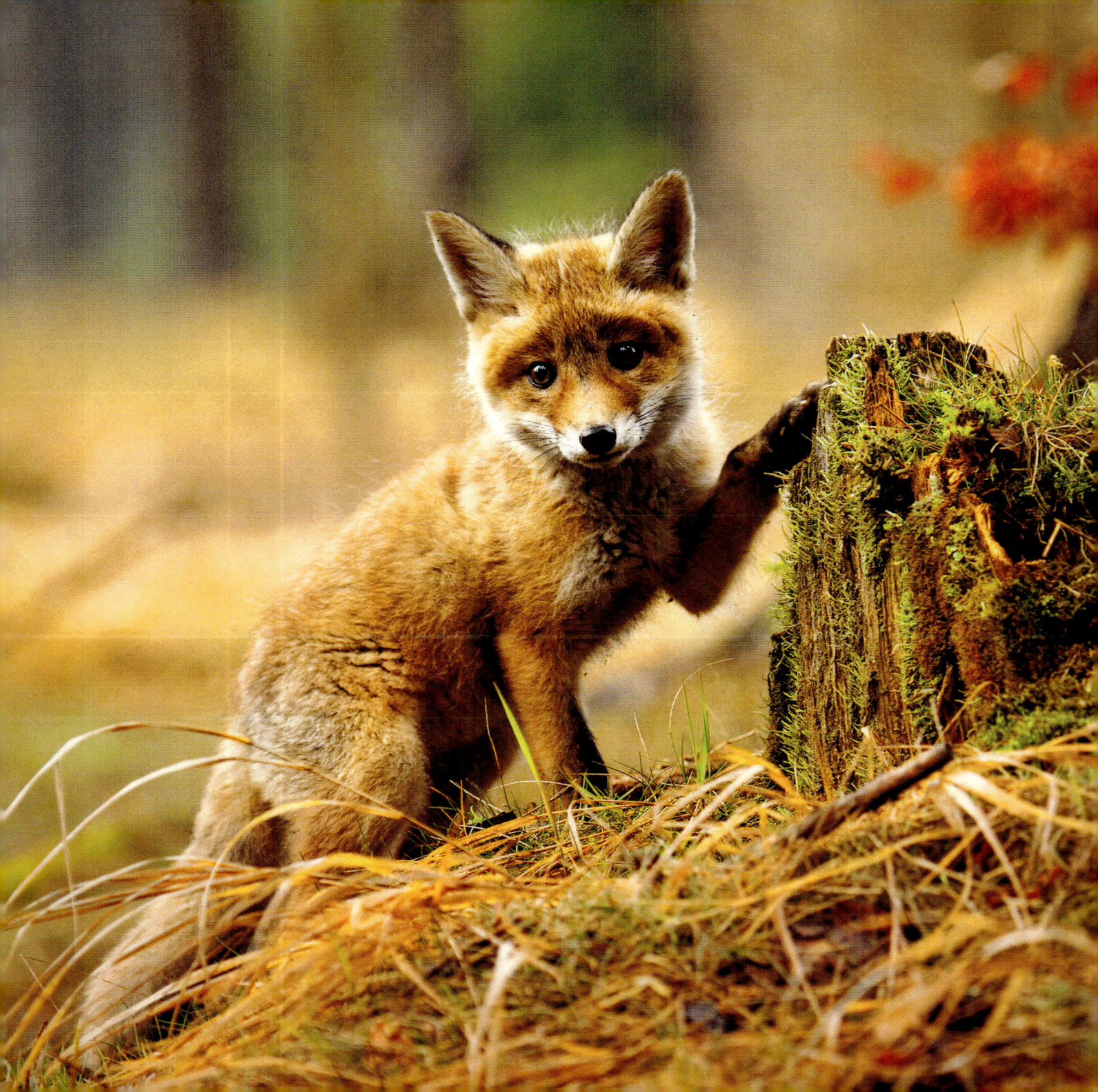

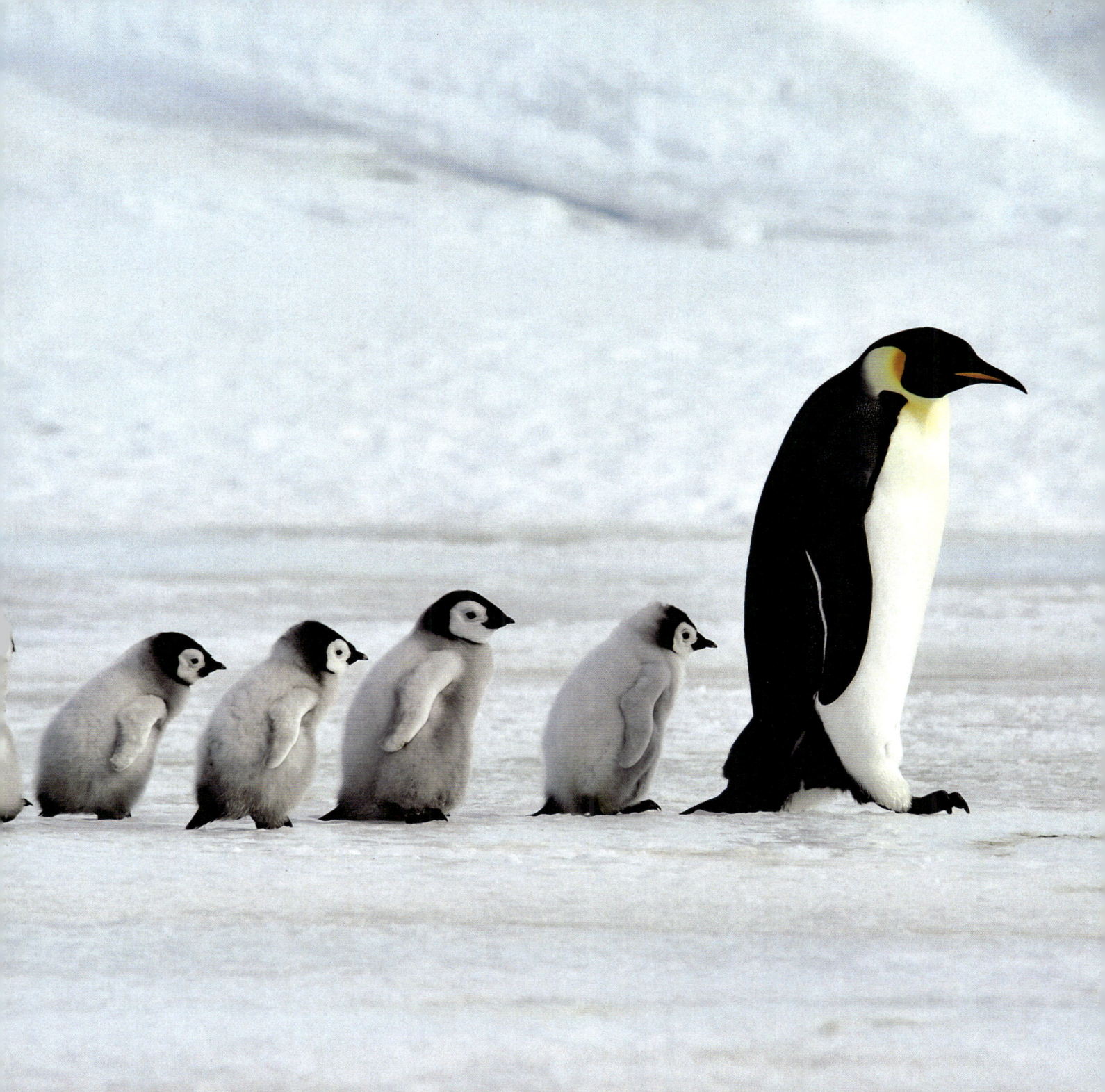

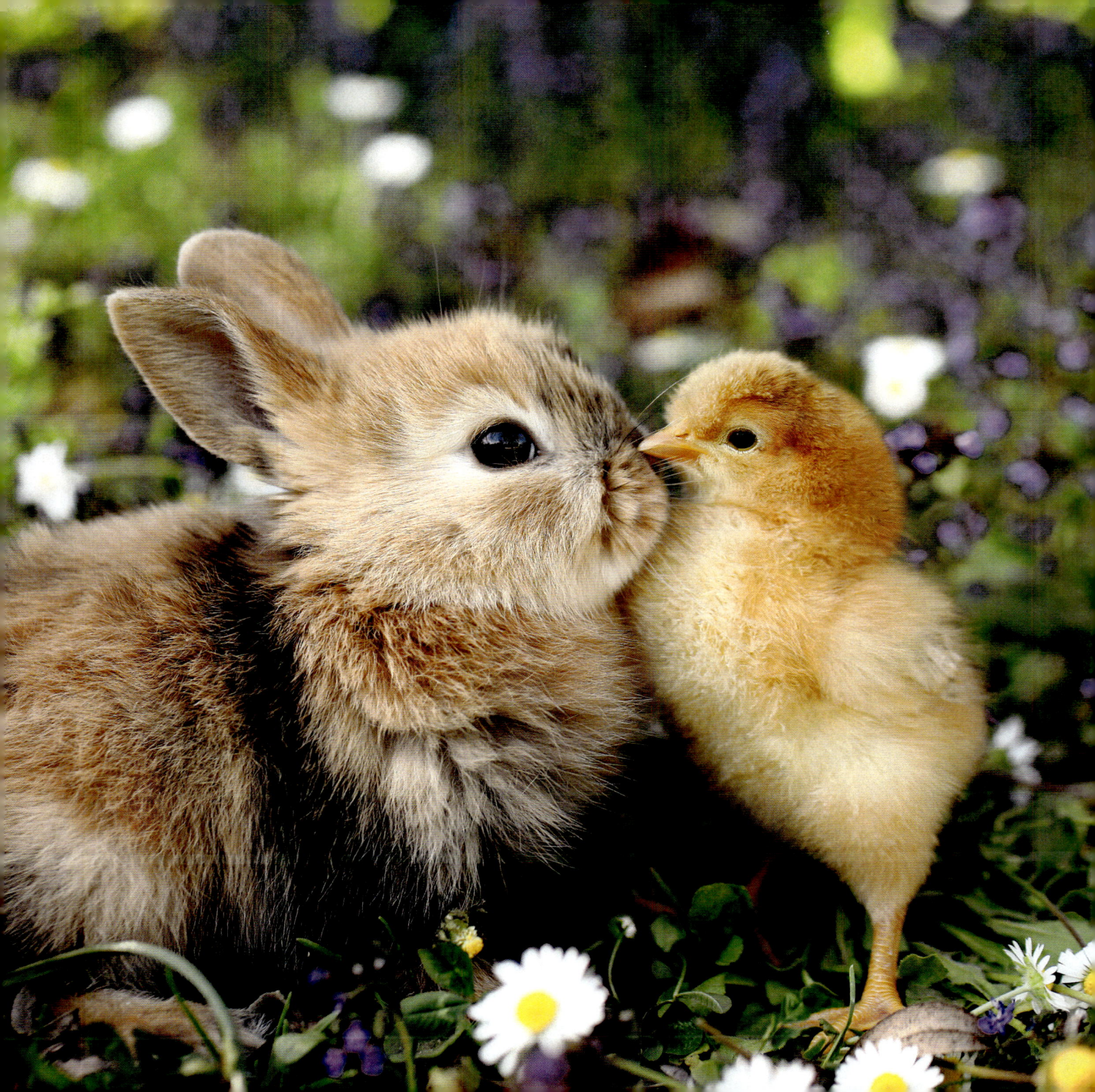

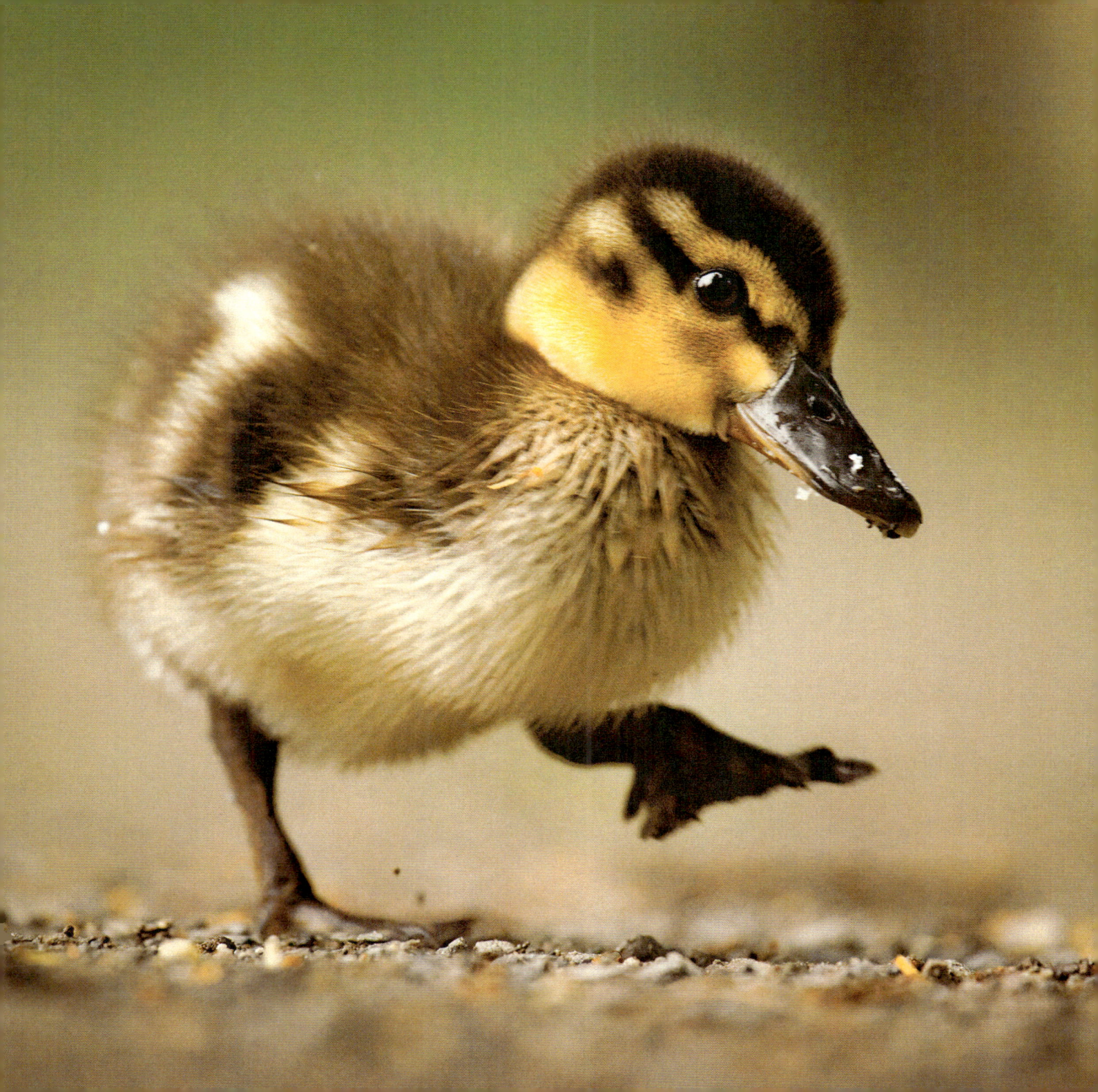

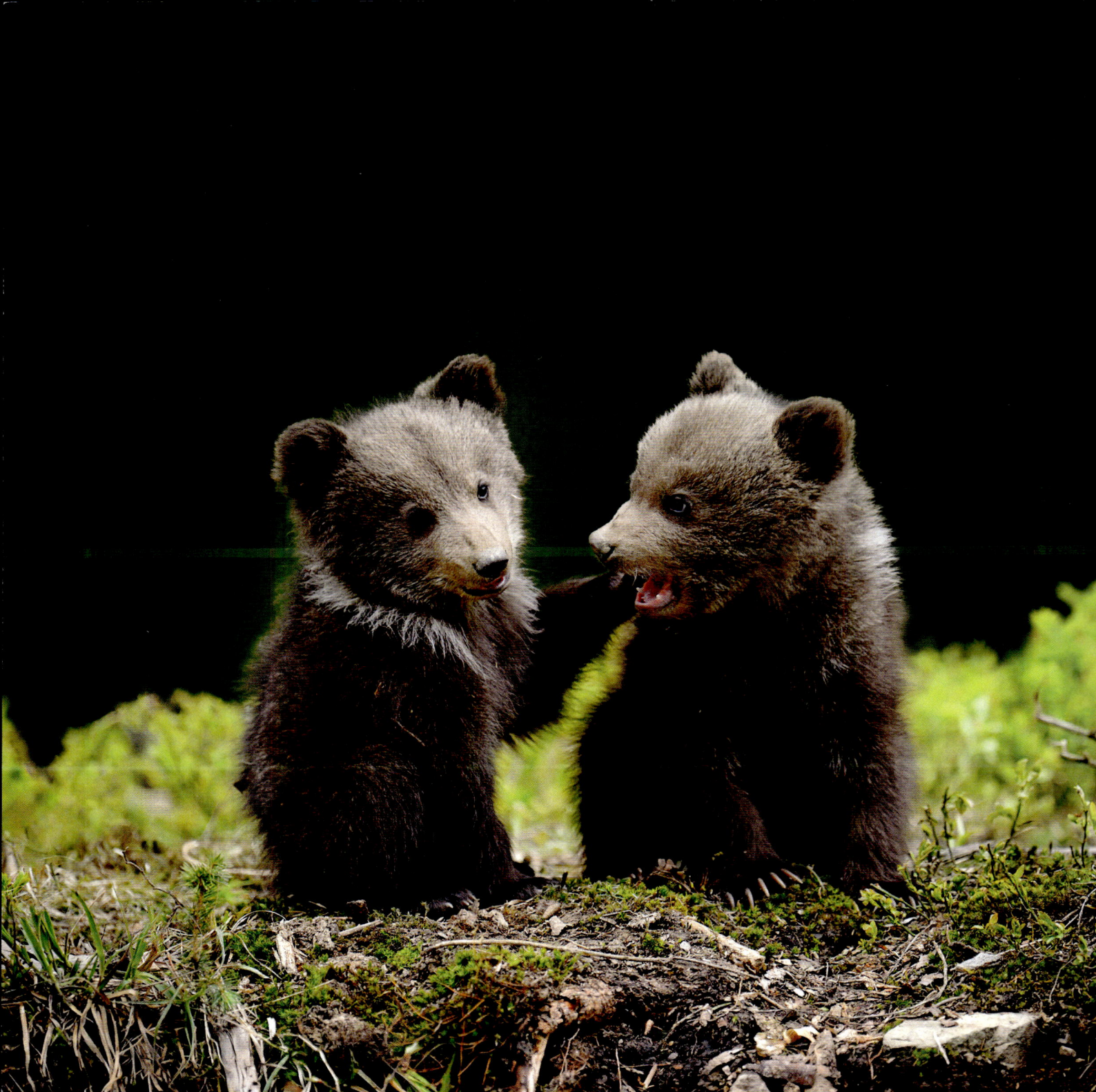

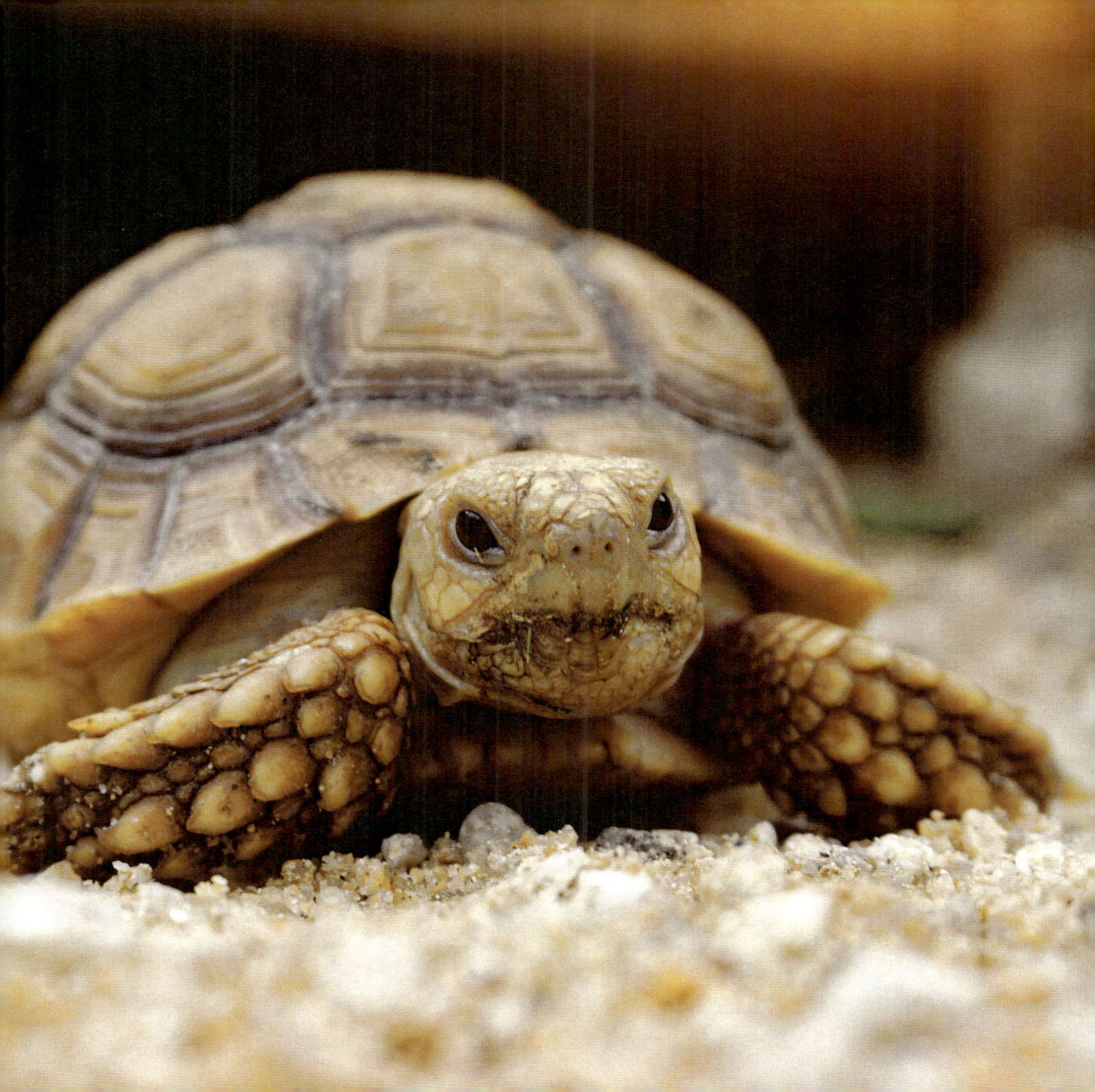

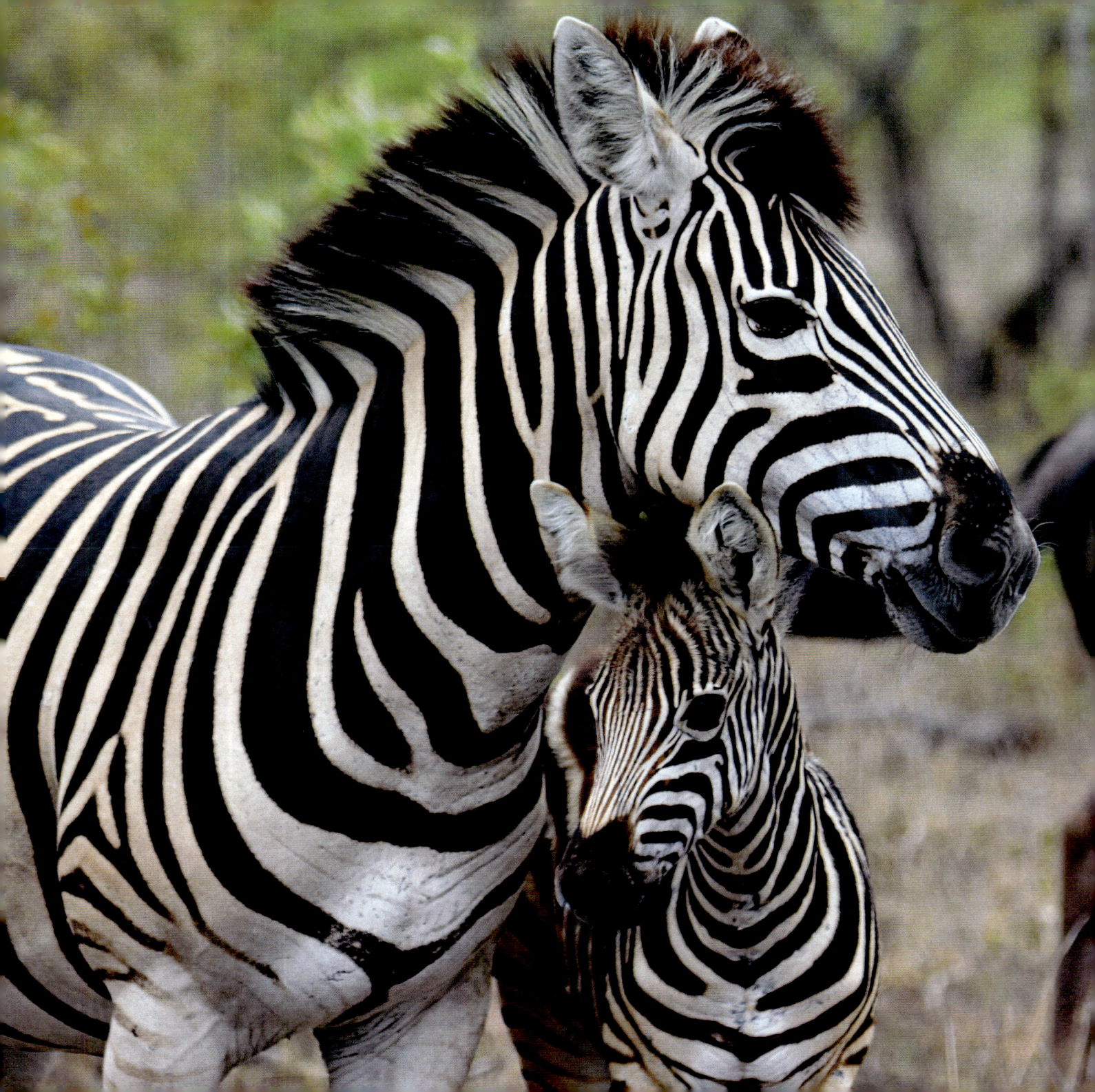

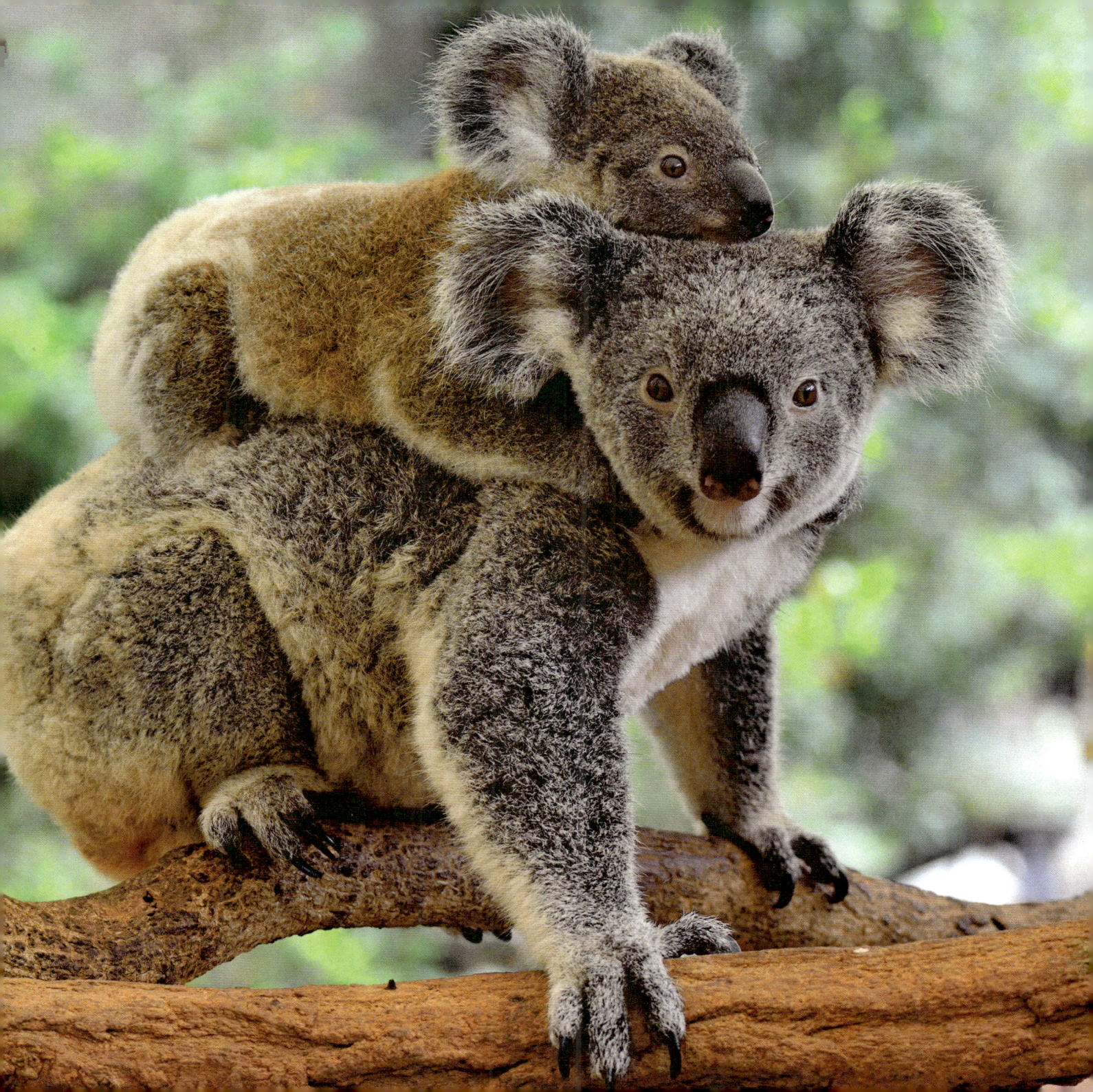

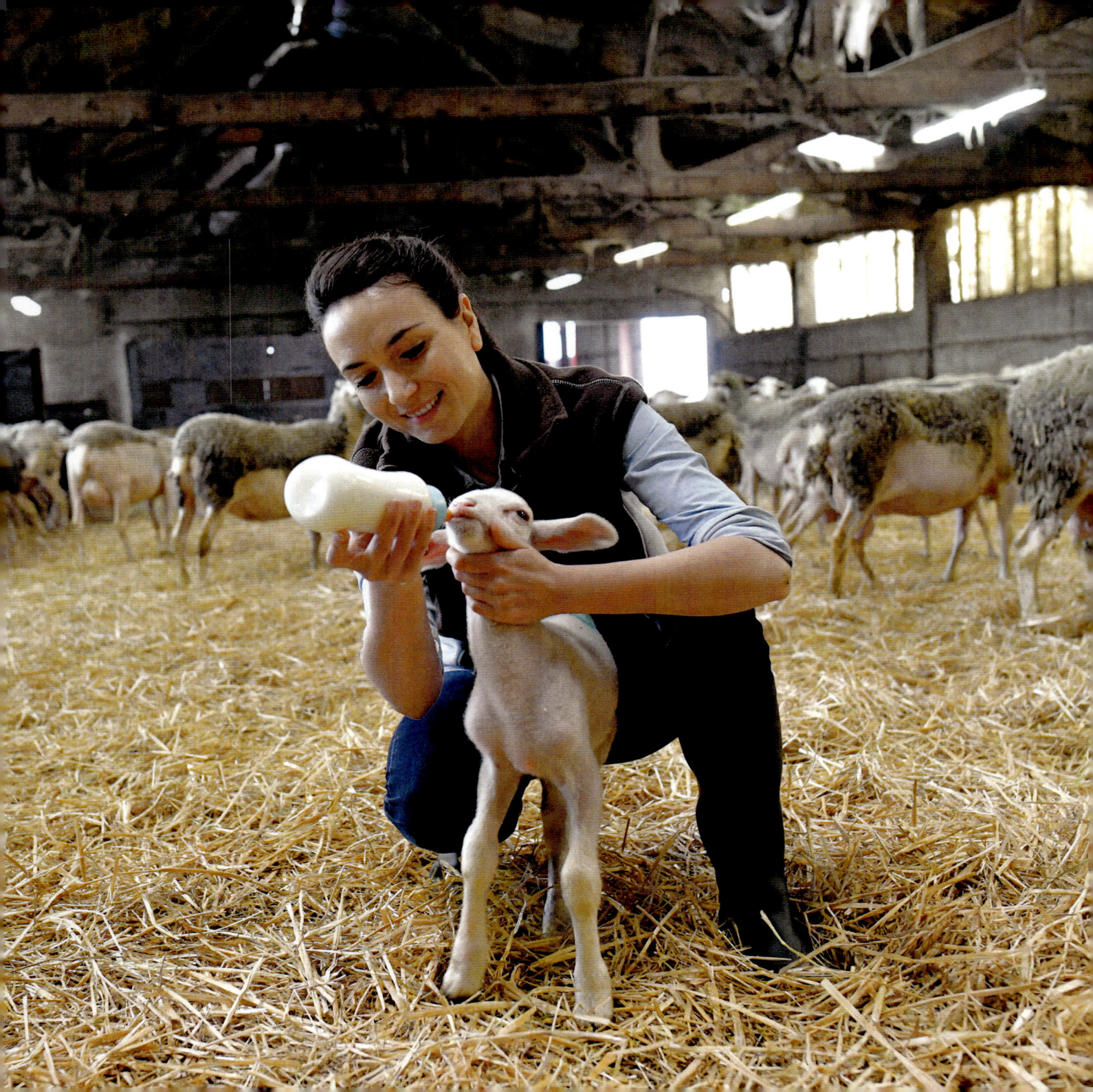

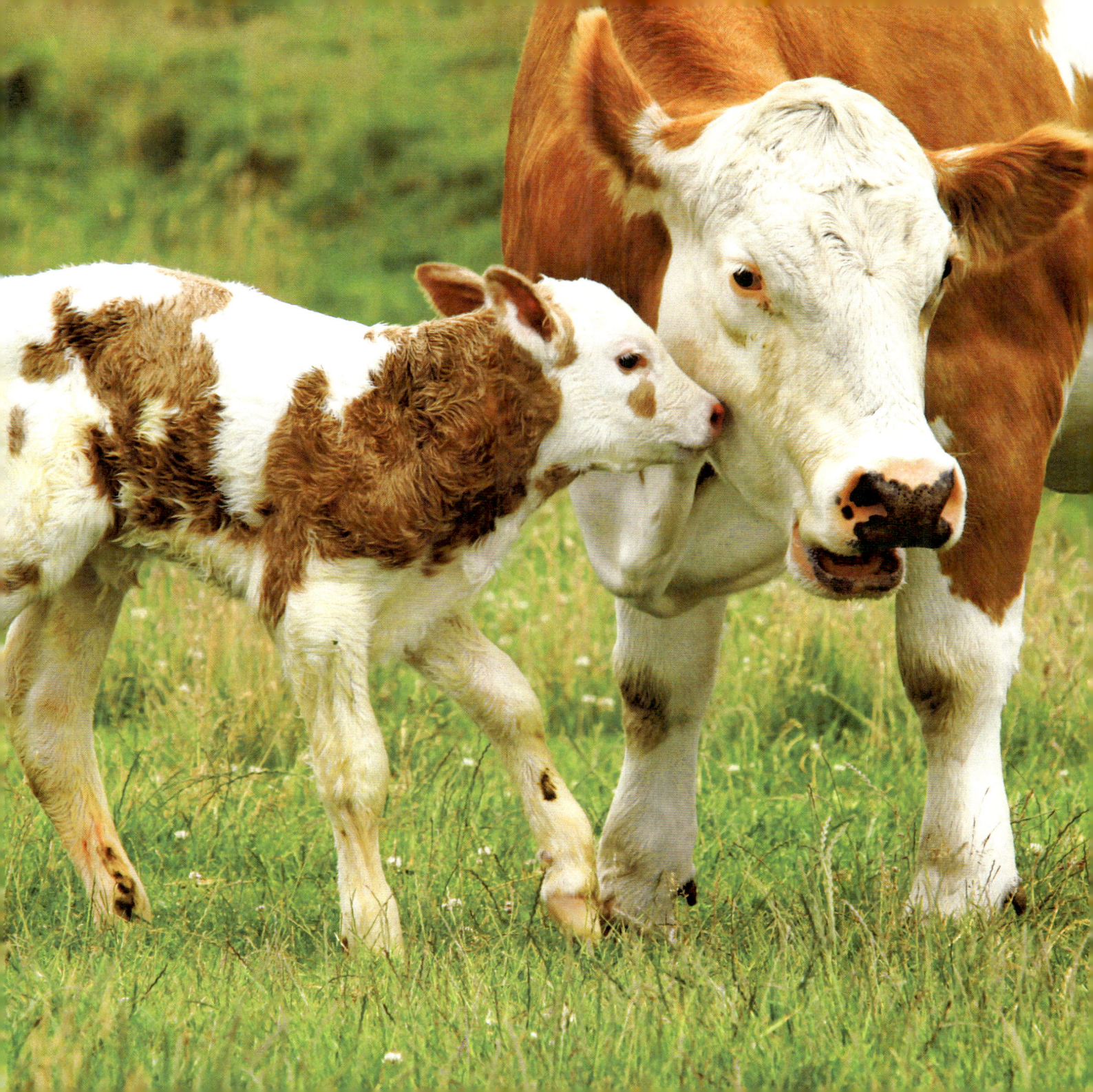

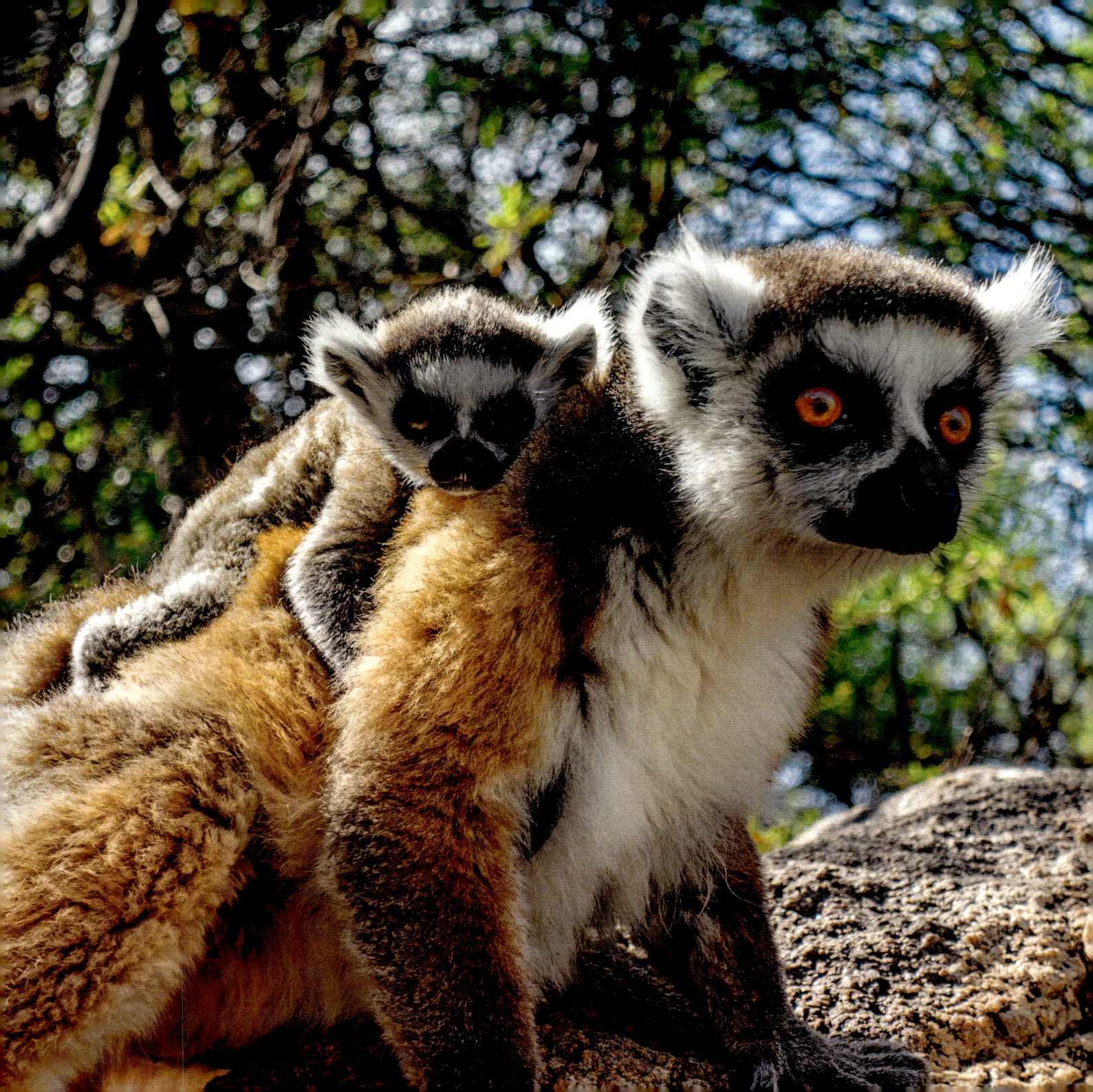

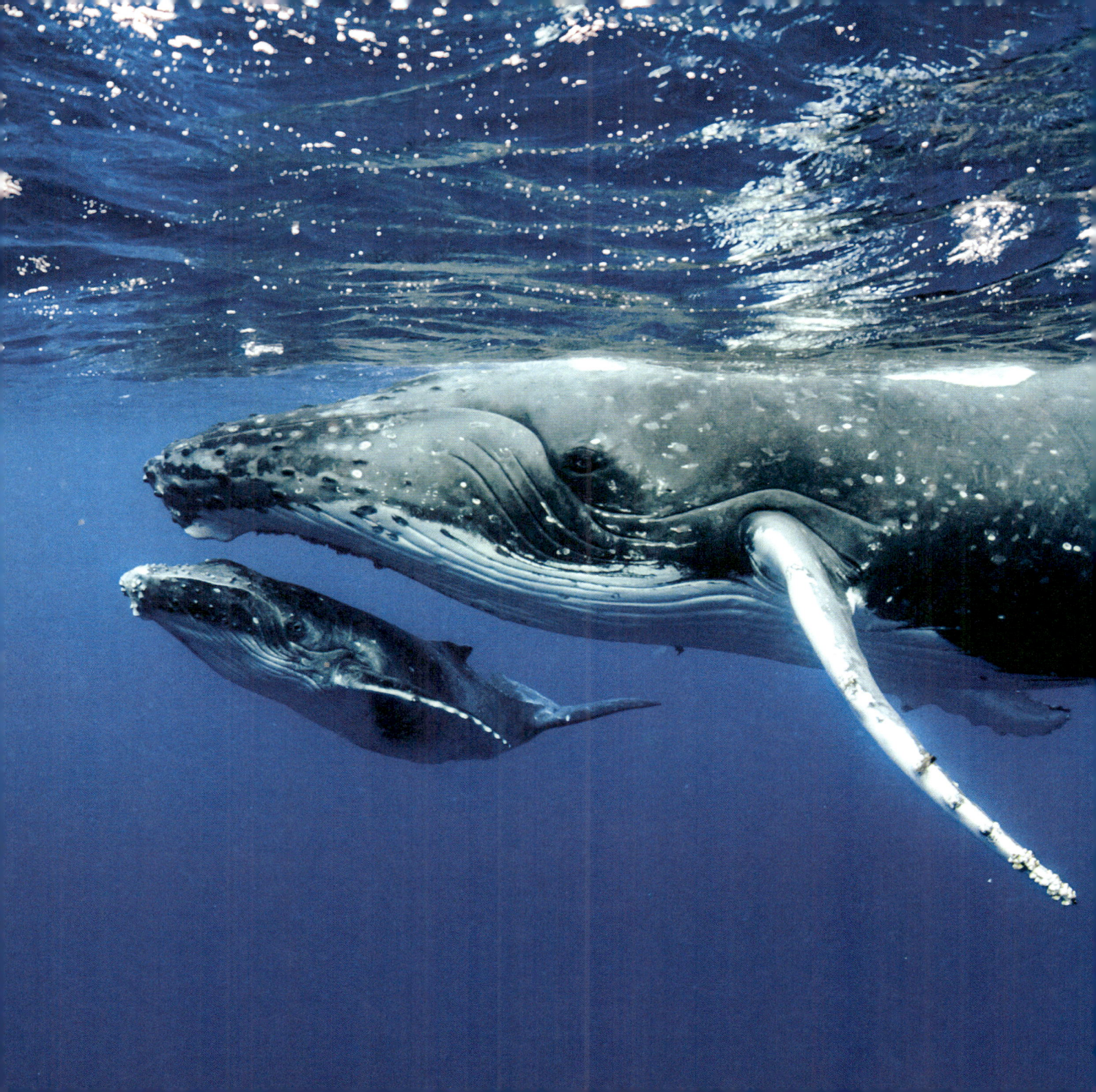

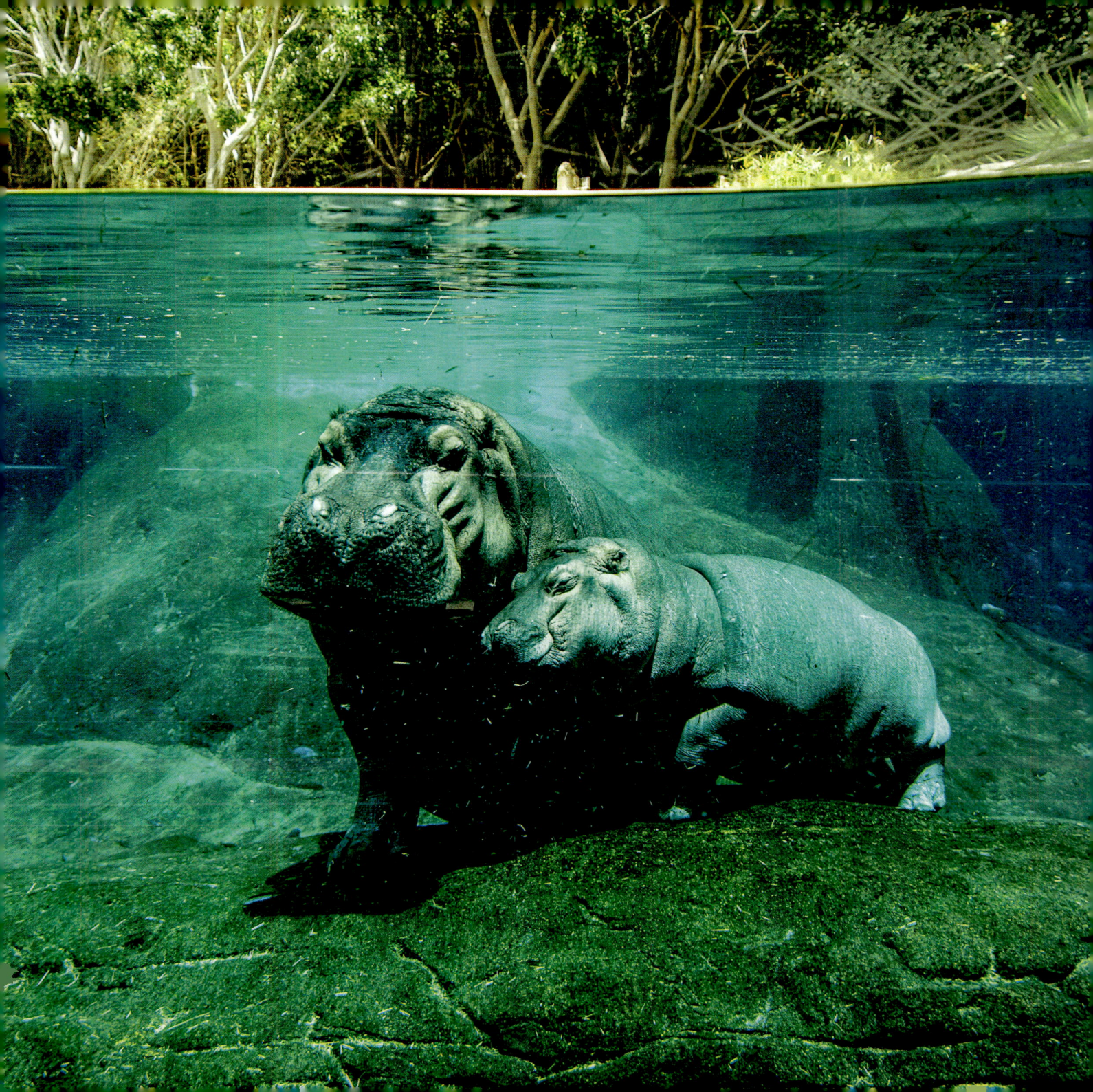

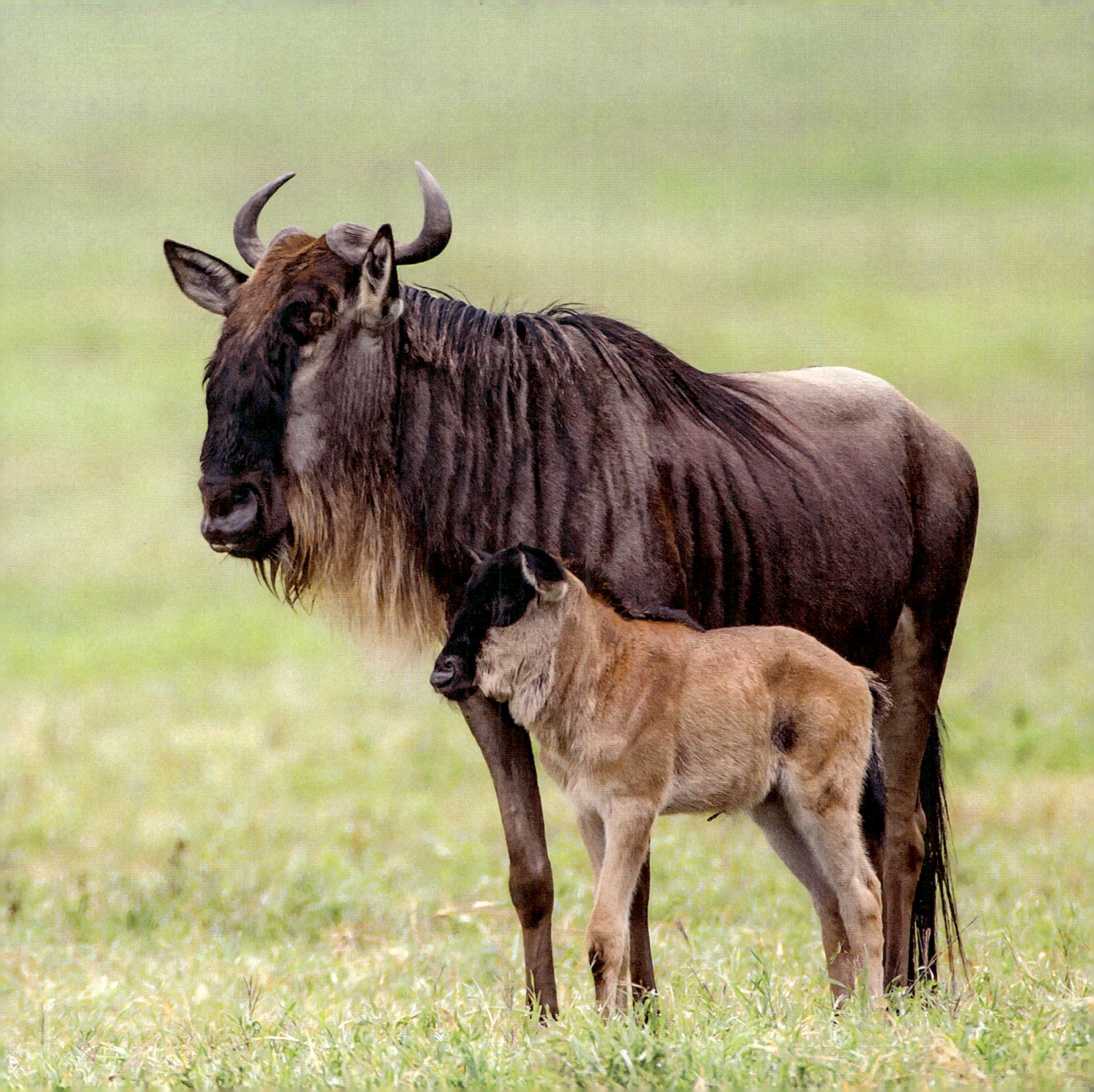

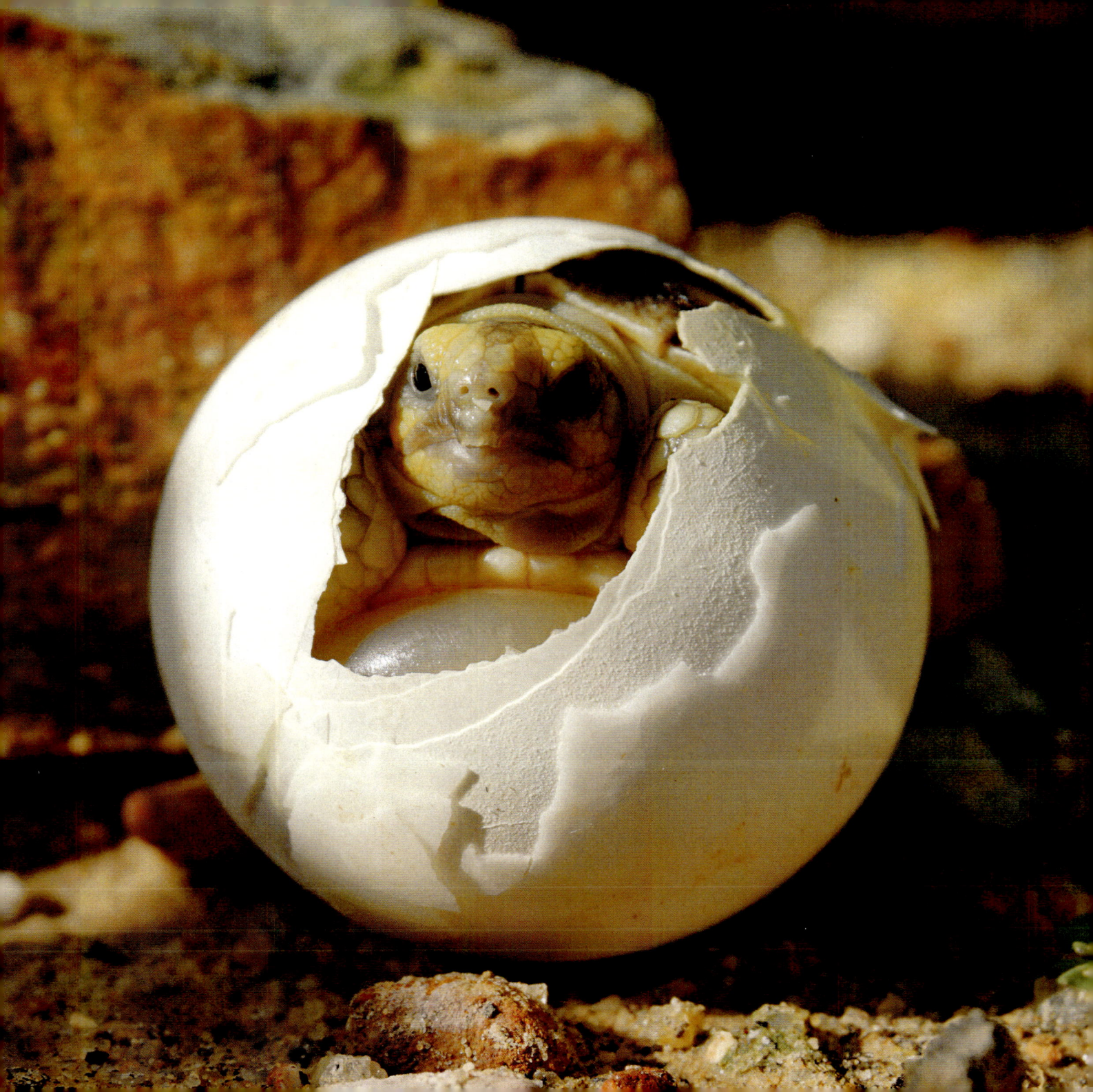

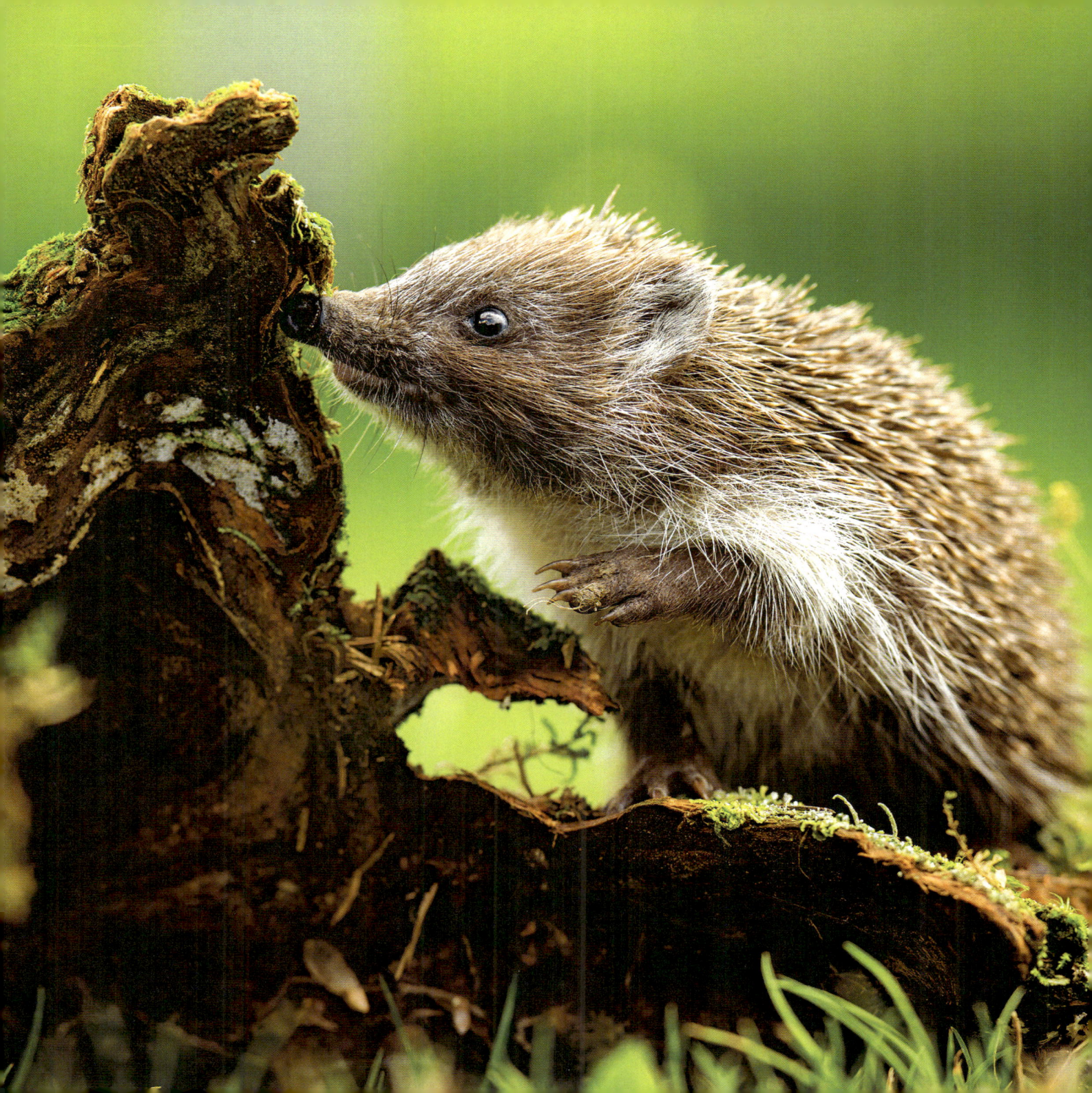

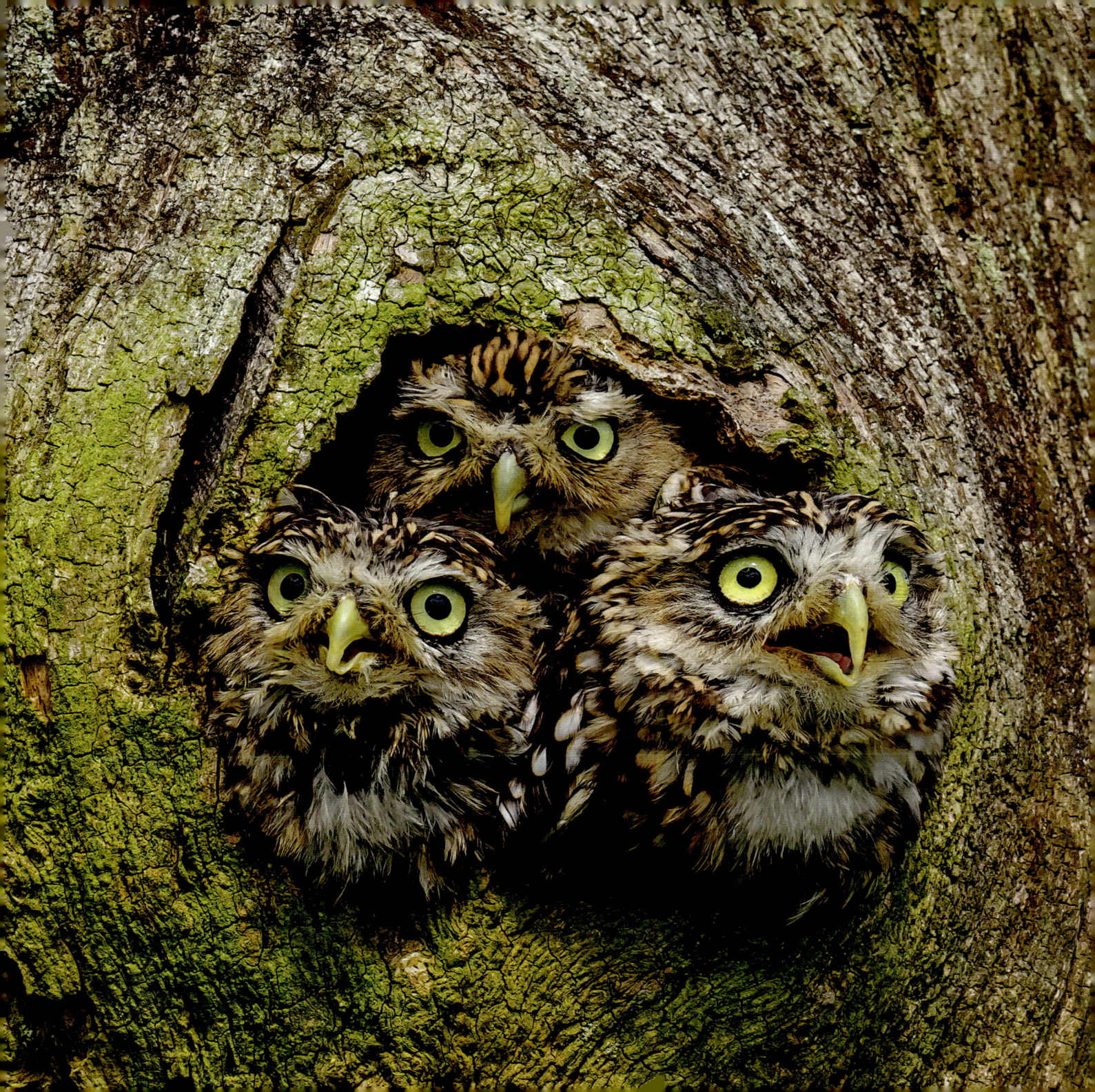

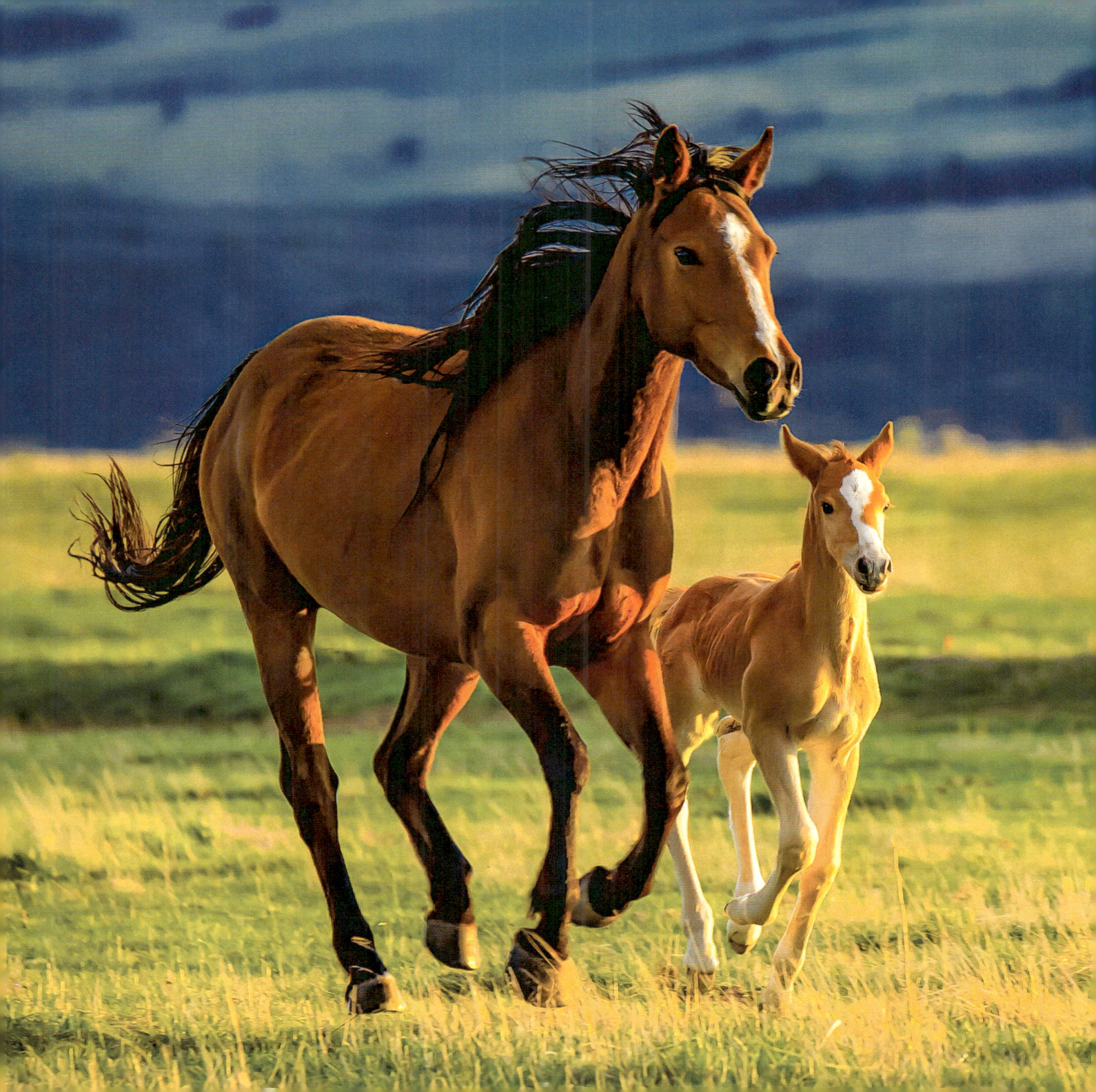

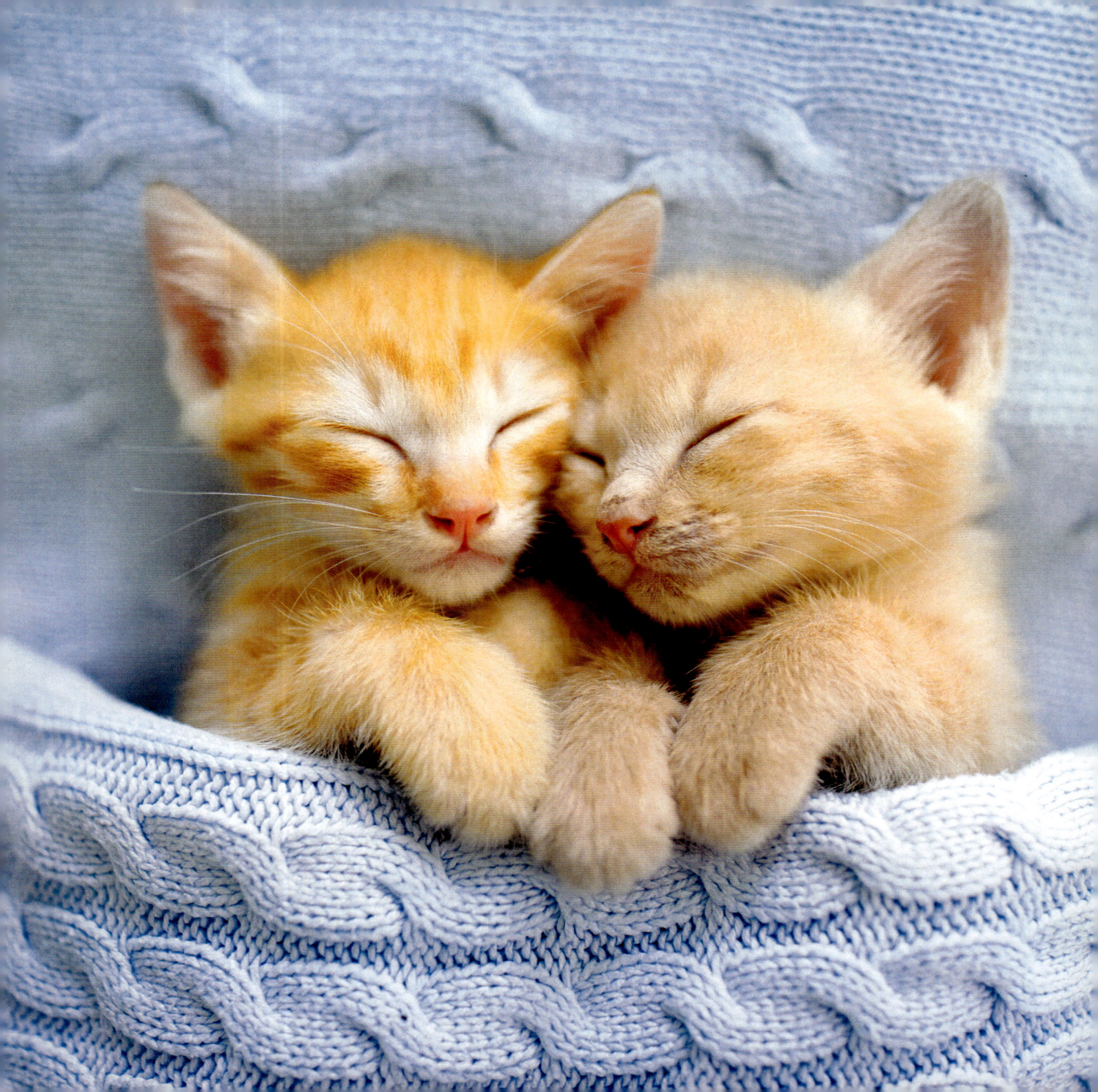

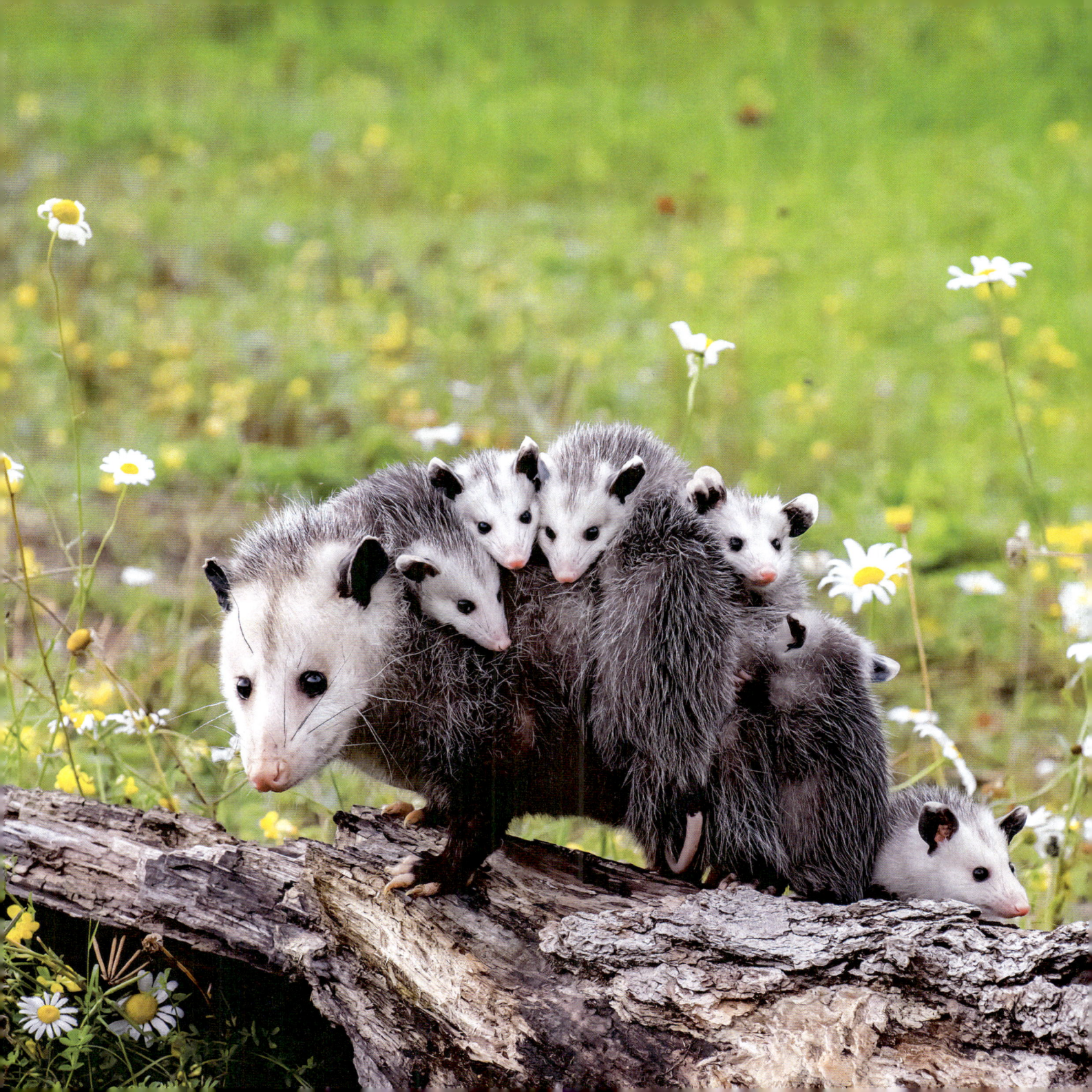

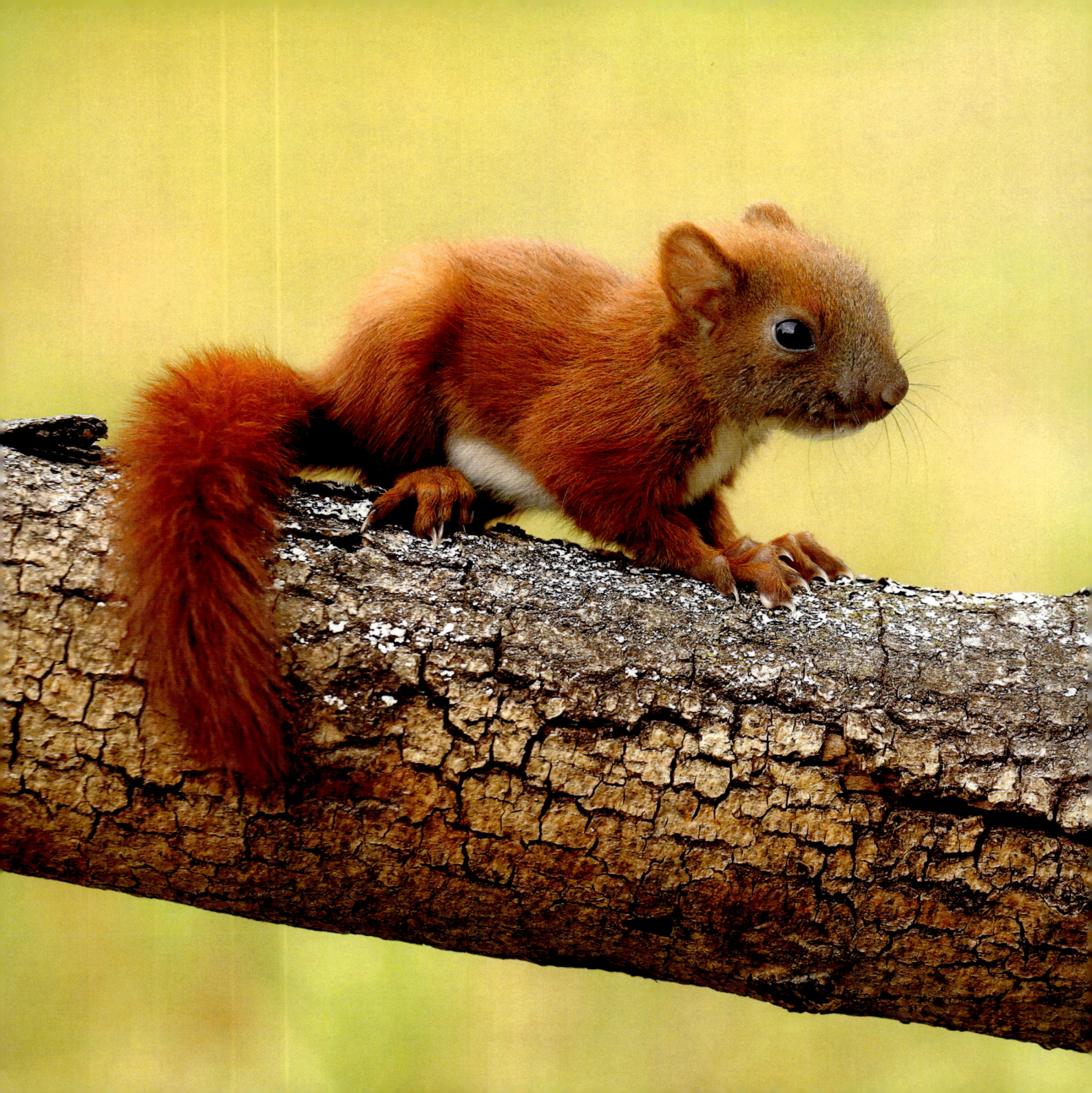

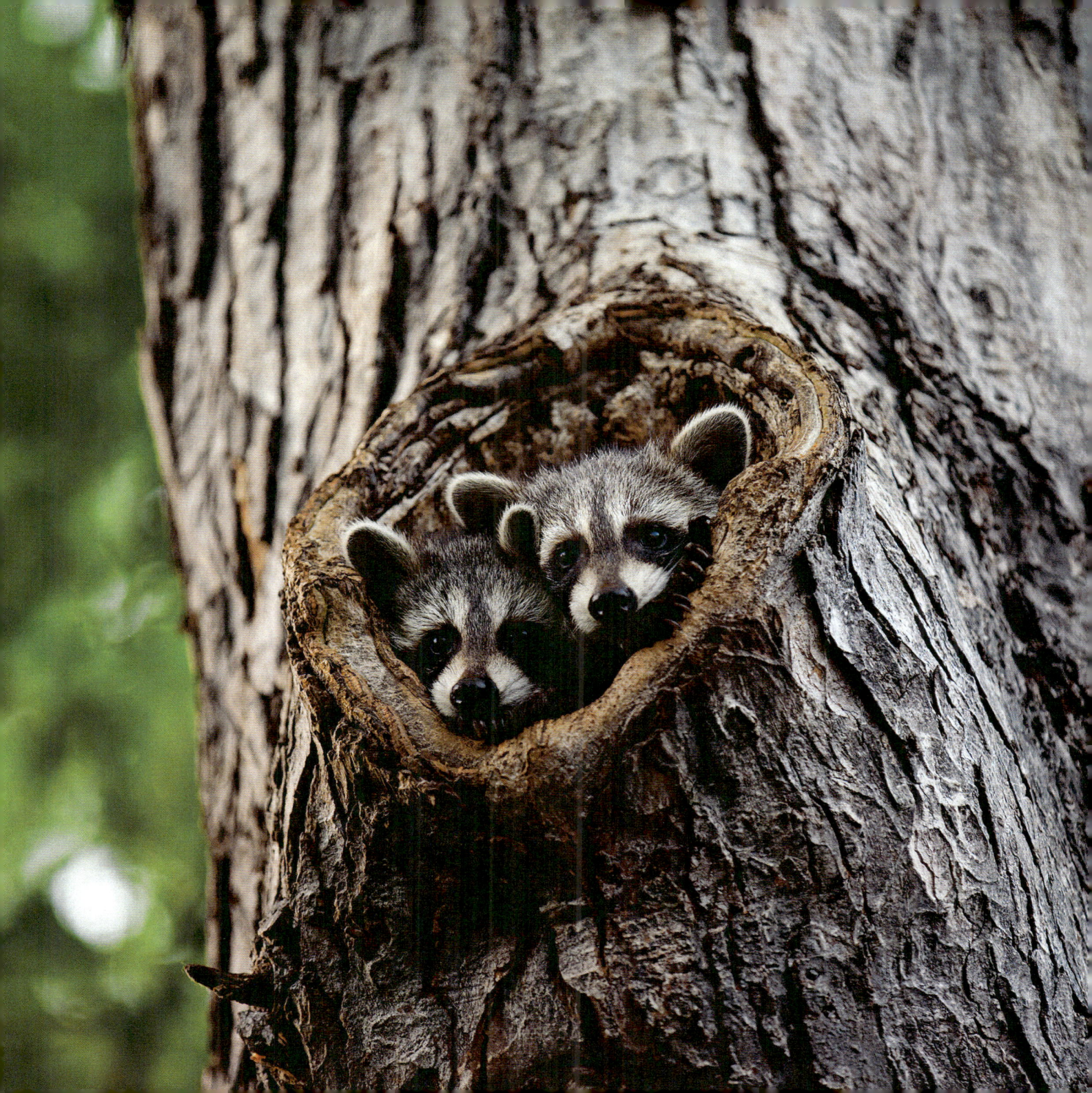

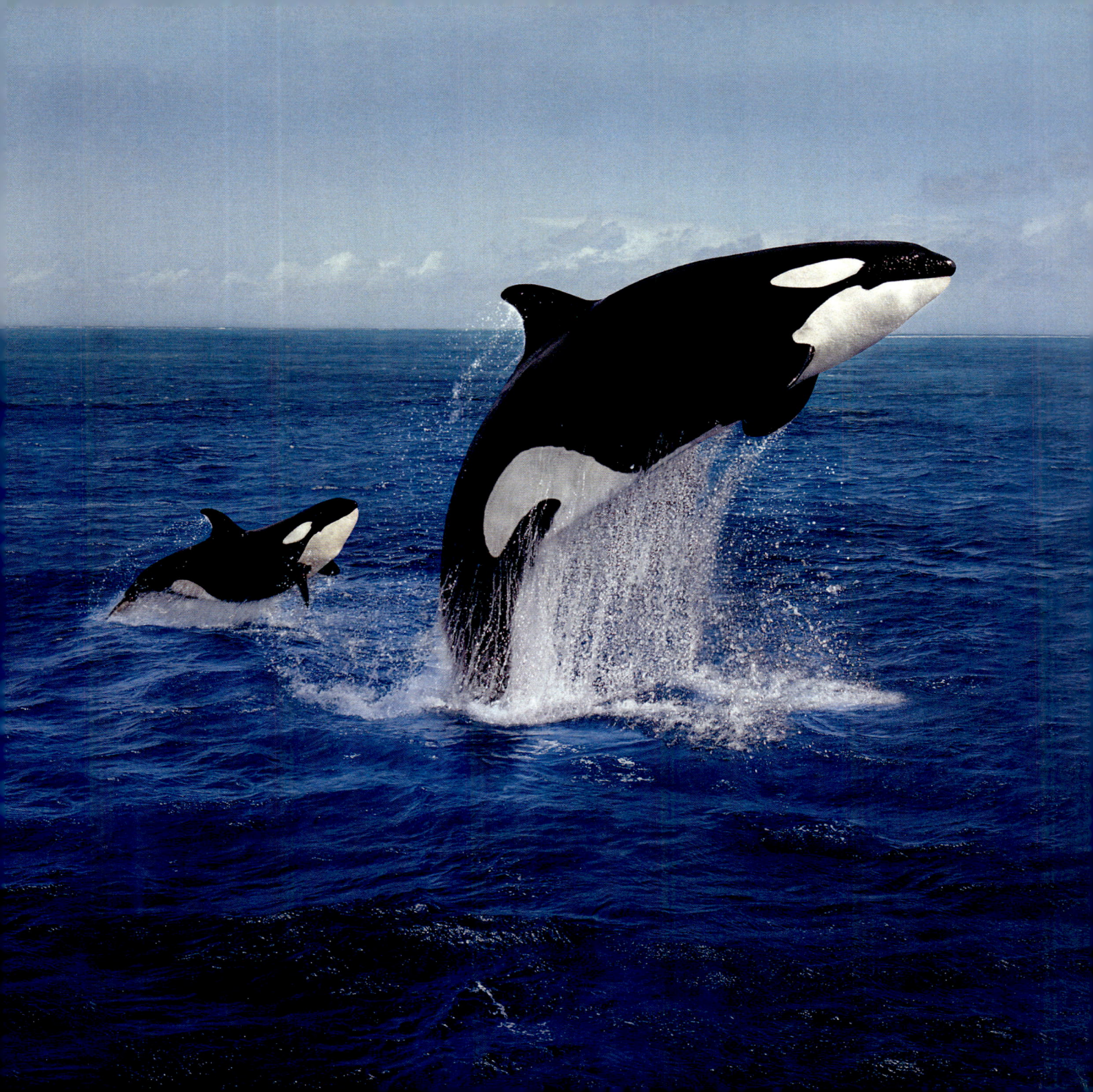

Made in United States
North Haven, CT
06 March 2022

16849714R00024